D0104165

Evidence-based Health Economics:

From effectiveness to efficiency in systematic review

Edited by

Cam Donaldson
Svare Chair in Health Economics, University of Calgary

Miranda Mugford
Professor of Health Economics, University of East Anglia

Luke Vale
Research Fellow, University of Aberdeen

BMJ Books

RA 410.5
.E956
2002

04904440Y

© BMJ Books 2002
BMJ Books is an imprint of the BMJ Publishing Group

All rights reserved. No part of this publication may be reproduced, stored in a retrieval system, or transmitted, in any form or by any means, electronic, mechanical, photocopying, recording and/or otherwise, without the prior written permission of the publishers.

First published in 2002
by BMJ Books, BMA House, Tavistock Square,
London WC1H 9JR

www.bmjbooks.com

British Library Cataloguing in Publication Data
A catalogue record for this book is available from the British Library

ISBN 0 7279 1579 7

Typeset by SIVA Math Setters, Chennai, India
Printed and bound in Spain by GraphyCems, Navarra

Contents

MAR 1 2 2003

Contributors

* denotes attendance at the Banff Workshop

Andre Ament* Associate Professor in Health Economics, Department of Health Organisation Policy and Economics, Faculty of Health Sciences, Maastricht University, Netherlands

Stephen Birch* Professor of Health Economics, Centre for Health Economics and Policy Analysis, McMaster University, Hamilton, Ontario, Canada

Paul Brown Senior Lecturer in Health Economics, Department of Community Health, University of Auckland, New Zealand

Douglas Coyle* Assistant Professor of Health Economics, Clinical Epidemiology Unit, Ottawa Health Research Institute, Ottawa Hospital; Departments of Medicine and Epidemiology and Community Medicine, University of Ottawa, Ontario, Canada

Gillian Currie* Assistant Professor of Economics, and Alberta Heritage Population Health Investigator, Departments of Economics and Community Health Sciences, University of Calgary; Fellow, Institute of Health Economics, Alberta, Canada

Vittorio Demicheli Cochrane Collaboration and Servizio Epidemiologia ASL 20, Alessandria, Italy

Henrica de Vet Associate Professor in Epidemiology, Institute for Research in Extramural Medicine, VU University Medical Centre, Amsterdam, Netherlands

Cam Donaldson* Svare Chair in Health Economics and Canadian Institutes of Health Research Senior Investigator, Departments of Community Health Sciences and Economics, University of Calgary; Fellow, Institute of Health Economics, Calgary, Alberta, Canada

Michael Drummond* Professor of Health Economics and Director, Centre for Health Economics, University of York, UK

Silvia Evers Postdoctoral Research Affiliate, Department of Health Organisation Policy and Economics, Faculty of Health Sciences, Maastricht University, Netherlands

Cindy Farquhar* Associate Professor in Reproductive Medicine, Cochrane Menstrual Disorders and Subfertility Group, National Women's Hospital, University of Auckland, New Zealand

Marielle Goossens Postdoctoral Research Affiliate, Institute for Rehabilitation Research, Hoensbroek and Maastricht University, Netherlands

Toby Gosden* Research Fellow, National Primary Care Research and Development Centre, University of Manchester, UK

Tom Jefferson* Cochrane Collaboration and Health Reviews Ltd, Rome, Italy

Ivar Sønbø Kristiansen* Associate Professor of Community Medicine, Institute of Public Health – Health Economics, University of Southern Denmark, Odense, Denmark

Karen M Lee Caro Research, Boston, Massachusetts, USA

Braden Manns* Assistant Professor of Medicine, Departments of Medicine and Community Health Sciences, University of Calgary; Fellow, Institute of Health Economics, Alberta, Canada

Miranda Mugford* Professor of Health Economics, School of Medicine, Health Policy and Practice, University of East Anglia, Norwich, UK

Luke Vale* Research Fellow, Health Economics Research Unit and Health Services Research Unit, University of Aberdeen, UK

Maurits van Tulder Epidemiologist, Senior Investigator HTA, Institute for Research in Extramural Medicine and Department of Clinical Epidemiology and Biostatistics, VU University Medical Centre, Amsterdam, Netherlands

Preface

Decision makers, when weighing up evidence, have to consider information produced from health economics, evidence-based medicine and systematic reviews. Despite their importance, these three sources of information are rarely considered together.

One attempt to do so was the formation of the Economics Methods Group within the Cochrane Collaboration in 1998. The Cochrane Economics Methods Group (CEMG) aims to

- Develop and disseminate methods for reviewing trials, and other studies, with economic elements, and for building economic evaluations from reviews of effectiveness.
- Be a discussion and methods development group for economists involved with Cochrane Reviews, to encourage transparency of methods and liaison with other methods groups on topics of common interest.
- Provide links for Cochrane Review Groups with health economists and other sources.
- Run workshops and discussions on economic issues and methods relevant to the aims of the Cochrane Collaboration.

Much of the work of the CEMG over the past three years has been in encouraging the collaboration of health economists and systematic reviewers. Many such joint ventures also take place outwith the auspices of the Cochrane Collaboration. It is important, therefore, to summarise the "state of the art" on how studies involving such collaborations are conducted. However, to improve such studies in the future, further research has to be carried out.

This book attempts to provide the reader with the underlying principles, along with case studies, of how to use systematic review data in economic evaluations. In doing this, it will be seen that different approaches can be used, each of which provides different results. This, in itself, sets an agenda for future research, to identify whether there is a best method, and, if so, what it is. The volume also provides challenges to the current evidence-based medicine paradigm, which permits us to rethink our overall approach to the use of evidence and economics in health policy making, and, again, provides us with food for future research.

The chapters in the book were initially presented as papers at a workshop, held at the Banff Centre for Continuing Education, Alberta, Canada in

February 2001. We would like to acknowledge the support, financial and otherwise, for this workshop provided by the Institute of Health Economics and its Chief Executive Officer, Dev Menon. We would also like to acknowledge the support of Mary Banks from BMJ Books, and Lindsay Bradshaw and Diane Lorenzetti of the University of Calgary for organising the production of the material.

Many unnamed colleagues have contributed informally through comments on drafts or discussions, and we thank them all. All three editors and other contributors acknowledge the support of their home institutions and funding bodies. We also thank Elsevier Science Ltd for permission to reproduce Figure 1.1.

Having mapped out current approaches and future directions for research, we hope that the book provides an exciting agenda for research and collaboration in this important area over the coming years.

Cam Donaldson
Miranda Mugford
Luke Vale

Co-convenors, Cochrane Economics Methods Group

1: From effectiveness to efficiency: an introduction to evidence-based health economics

CAM DONALDSON, MIRANDA MUGFORD,
LUKE VALE

Introduction

Evidence-based medicine (EBM) has become synonymous with the notion of systematic reviews. Such systematic reviews attempt to assemble data, from published and unpublished sources, on the effectiveness of health care interventions. The aim has been to inform clinical practice and, of course, to change practice where patient and public health can be improved.

However, evidence-based practice isolated from economic issues is not realistic, and, indeed, may ultimately harm patients and the public. More fundamentally, narrow evidence-based medicine methodologies may themselves contribute to inefficient health policy and greater inequalities in health. Evidence-based health economics recognises not only the need for the use of evidence-based principles in economic evaluation but also that such principles should themselves be based on economics concepts.

Therefore, in this book, the intention is to:

- discuss the role of systematic reviews in economic evaluations of health care;
- provide case studies to demonstrate how systematic reviews can be used in economic evaluations; and
- show the limitations of current evidence-based approaches and how economics can be used to improve and broaden the evidence base in ways that are more relevant for policy makers.

In this introductory chapter, it is important to consider, first, the importance of economics to systematic review. This is reinforced by reflecting on the views of two of the founding fathers of evidence-based medicine and health economics – Archie Cochrane and Alan Williams. The chapter goes on from there to outline the limitations of evidence-based medicine and a health economics approach built on such foundations, and introduce a conceptual framework for the book. This introduction is illustrated with examples of policy questions that can be addressed by an evidence-based health economics approach. Finally, the contents of the book are outlined in more detail.

The importance of economics in systematic review

The main purpose of systematic reviews of health care interventions has been seen as providing information about the effectiveness of these interventions.[1] Typically, systematic reviews in EBM are designed to test a hypothesis as to whether a new form of health care is or is not more effective than an alternative, using dichotomous measures, via odds ratios or relative risks, rather than continuous measures, such as effect size. These reviews are not usually designed to ask the question "how much more effective is the new form of care". The issue of how to estimate effect size is central to Chapter 5, by Coyle and Lee.

In order to judge how to act on the evidence from systematic reviews in the face of scarce resources, decision makers need to consider further evidence. Nearly every health care intervention has an impact not only on health and social welfare but also on the resources used in the production of care. As resources have alternative beneficial uses and as different people may place different values on the various health outcomes, then, to make the best decisions about alternative courses of action, information is needed on the health benefits and also the extent of resource use (or cost) of these courses of action.

The need to assess the "economic" gain from alternative forms of care is reflected in the continuing development of economic evaluation methods and the increasing numbers of studies with health economic input. Compilers of clinical practice guidelines are also placing more emphasis on economic data.[2] Economic evaluations of interventions are central to informing the advice and decisions issued by organisations such as the UK's National Institute for Clinical Excellence (NICE) and the Australian Government's Pharmaceutical Benefits Advisory Committee (PBAC). That is, these organisations are concerned with issues of cost-effectiveness and cost-benefit. When addressing such issues, the types of policy question that can be addressed are:

- "For a given group of patients, is drug X more effective and less costly than current treatment?" or
- "For a given group of patients, is drug Y more costly as well as more effective than current treatment, and, if so, what are the magnitudes of the extra costs and effectiveness?" or
- "Because drug Y is more costly than current treatment, if we are considering implementing drug Y, from where would the resources come, and is this change worth making in terms of the benefits given up?"

Reviewers for bodies such as NICE and PBAC are finding that more trials now include an economic element, and there is an increasing need for guidance about judging the quality of economic evaluation, reporting the outcomes and summarising the results. One of the foremost organisations in the pursuit of rigorous evidence on the effectiveness of interventions is the Cochrane Collaboration – an international organisation with the aim of improving the effectiveness of health care throughout the world by preparing, maintaining and making accessible systematic reviews of the effects of health care. Although health technology and pharmaceutical regulation bodies do not all take the same approach, they are all interested in best evidence. In this book, the focus is on systematic review as defined by the Cochrane Collaboration, whereby the primary source of that evidence is data from randomised trials and other types of robust study. We begin, therefore, by making the case that Archie Cochrane, who inspired much of the systematic review movement (and of course the Cochrane Collaboration), was in favour of decisions in health care being made on the basis of evidence on economics as well as effectiveness. To do this, we have turned to the published reflections of a person who has inspired much of the "health economics movement" over the past 30 years – Alan Williams of the University of York.

Cochrane, Williams and health economics

In his 1998 Cochrane Lecture, Alan Williams describes how Archie Cochrane changed his life.[3] However, it is not difficult to see that Cochrane was also influenced by Williams, who acted as an Economic Advisor to the Treasury and what was then known as the Department of Health and Social Security (DHSS) in England in the 1960s. At that time, Cochrane was a leading academic medical researcher, with close ties to the DHSS. The title of Cochrane's most famous work, his book of Rock Carling lectures, is *Effectiveness* ***and Efficiency*** … [our emphasis].[4] The box below contains two quotations from that book, illustrating the importance that Cochrane placed on economics.

Archie Cochrane on health economics

"Allocations of funds and facilities are nearly always based on the opinions of senior consultants, but, more and more, requests for additional facilities will have to be based on detailed arguments with 'hard evidence' as to the gain to be expected from the patients' angle **and the cost.** Few can possibly object to this."[4] (p. 82)

"If we are ever going to get the 'optimum' results from our national expenditure on the NHS we must finally be able to express the results in the form of the benefit **and the cost** to the population of a particular type of activity, and the increased benefit that would be obtained if more money were made available."[4] (p. 2)

If a goal is to make systematic reviews of effectiveness more relevant, it could be argued that Cochrane's quotes reflect the sentiment that considerations of resource use can do this. That is, considering cost-effectiveness (or efficiency) is more important than considering clinical excellence (or effectiveness) alone. To consider efficiency, we have to link data on costs and benefits of care and we have to accept that decisions made on the basis of such information will, either explicitly or implicitly, involve valuations of human life, pain and suffering.

Archie Cochrane's early support for a National Health Service in the UK is well known. However, he was equally passionate in his belief that an NHS should deliver only beneficial care to patients. Thus, he is famous for having modified a banner which originally read "All care should be free!" to "All *effective* care should be free!" Williams convinces us, from his reading of Cochrane's work and given the plethora of (effective) interventions that could be funded by a modern health care system, that Cochrane would have further amended his banner to read "All *cost-effective* care should be free!"[3]

Taking that as Cochrane's basic motto, how do we go about compiling the best evidence on the economics of interventions in addition to documenting their effectiveness? Can the approach outlined aid with reviewing evidence on health and health care policy more broadly? What are the limitations of the approach?

The limitations of evidence-based medicine and economic evaluation

Maynard has criticised evidence-based medicine for considering only effectiveness of treatments and not their costs, as well as for not considering issues related to equity.[5] The former criticism has been dealt with above. On the latter, there are likely to be cases where poorer people have greater

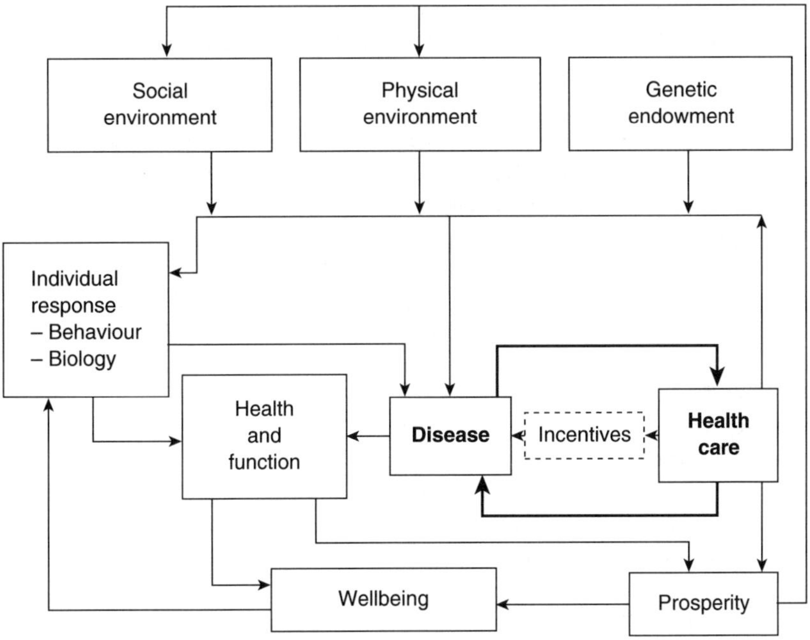

Figure 1.1 Evans and Stoddart's determinants-of-health model.

capacity to benefit from limited resources and, thus, efficiency and equity coincide. However, the point Maynard makes is that we may decide to forgo efficiency (maximising health gains) in favour of allocating some resources to poorer people who have less capacity to benefit. Poorer people, if treated, may not do as well on average as those who are better off, but this may still be a trade-off we are willing to make.

This highlights the need for a broader perspective on evidence-based medicine and economic evaluation. For example, consider the determinants-of-health framework constructed by Evans and Stoddart,[6] replicated here in Figure 1.1. In the core of this model, in the emboldened boxes, health care impacts on disease and the need for health care is determined by disease. This relationship forms much of the focus of evidence-based medicine. However, as can be seen from the wider model, there are many sources of impact on disease, and hence on health and wellbeing. Focusing on these boxes raises a whole new set of policy questions which can be addressed, such as:

- "What is it about people's environments and social status that makes some more healthy than others?" or
- "What is it about people's environments and social status that results in some groups responding better to interventions than others?" or

- "For people with the same underlying clinical problem, should we be designing different interventions for people with different environmental and social backgrounds?"

These questions are rarely addressed in an evidence-based medicine paradigm, but should be considered by an evidence-based health economics approach in which we are trying to provide the most effective and equitable health care from available resources.

A further issue not taken into account in Figure 1.1 is the way health care is organised and funded. For example, the incentives engendered by different payment mechanisms will influence the amounts and types of health care provided. This, in turn, will impact, at least indirectly, on disease. To reflect this, note the addition of the box with a dotted border between those on health care and disease. An example of the types of policy question addressed in this box would be:

- "What is the impact on health outcomes and costs of remunerating physicians by different methods (such as salary versus fee-for-service)?"

This (slightly adapted) determinants-of-health model serves as a template for the remainder of the book. For the most part the book concentrates on the emboldened area. This is simply an extension of current approaches to systematic review and to economic evaluation. However, it will be seen that these current approaches become, at best, limited and, at worst, inappropriate, when considering issues of how to generate and use evidence to inform broader health policy. Different interventions and different types of research (for example, beyond the simple single intervention, patient based, randomised trial) may be required to inform this broader approach to determining health policy and to deciding how best to organise and finance our health care systems.

Overview of the book

Aims

Two of the aims of this book (introduced on page 1) consider how to incorporate economic evaluation into the process of systematic review or, conversely, how to include results of a systematic review in an economic evaluation. This is not straightforward. Therefore, this will be done by illustrating the state of the art in combining economic evaluations and systematic reviews; in particular, how the use of different methods can lead to different results and the lack of consensus on some important aspects of economic evaluation. The third major aim of the book is to highlight the limitations of evidence-based medicine and the contributions that economics can make to informing evidence-based health policy more generally. In meeting this aim, the focus is on assessing the evidence on *economic* interventions aimed at improving incentives in health care systems and on going beyond the comparison of health care interventions to comparisons of the health of socioeconomic groups and how these groups may respond differentially to interventions.

Content

The basic principles of the economic approach and how it relates to systematic review are outlined in Chapter 2 (Donaldson *et al*). This is then followed by two case studies (by Mugford in Chapter 3, and Farquhar and Brown in Chapter 4) in which it will be seen that in economic evaluations based on systematic reviews of effects of care, the approach is likely to involve use of data from sources other than the randomised trials included in the systematic review; for example, data on the baseline risks of the key outcomes (both health and resource use). Data on resource use and cost may also need to be informed by results from observational studies and primary data collection. This is not unusual. Indeed, even with economic evaluation alongside a randomised trial, some of the burden of data collection (for both costs and outcomes) quite legitimately falls outwith the trial.[7] However, it raises further questions about how to judge the quality of studies.

What is not clear, however, is which are the most appropriate sources for the different types of data required (resource use, prices, patient outcomes) to conduct the evaluation. Chapter 5 (Coyle and Lee) demonstrates how different results can arise from economic evaluations based on differences in the methods used to estimate costs and clinical effects of the interventions, whilst Chapters 6 to 8 examine issues of the difference made by using the best available evidence on effectiveness at the time of the economic evaluation and trends in the quality of economic evaluations over time in this regard (Jefferson *et al* and Demicheli *et al*) as well as the difficulties in achieving consensus amongst economists on the best approach to conducting economic evaluations alongside systematic reviews (Ament *et al*).

Finally, the economic contribution to evidence-based health policy does not stop at the economic evaluation of health care interventions. Moving into the box with the dotted boundary in Figure 1.1, many interventions are themselves economic. By this, it is meant that part of the solution to improving the health of the population may lie in having the incentives in place to encourage best practice. These incentives themselves require evaluation before their introduction. However, as will be seen in Chapter 9, by Kristiansen and Gosden, systematic review of evidence in this field is not as straightforward as in the case of evaluation of health care interventions. But it is still possible. The Cochrane Collaboration's EPOC (Effective Practice and Organisation of Care) Group has been compiling evidence on, amongst other things, such incentives.

Furthermore, the evaluation of interventions, based on the model of the randomised trial and other controlled comparisons, may mask important contributory factors to the health of populations. This is because such factors will be equalised across groups in a well designed trial. However, the key to an evidence-based health policy may lie in what we can learn about the degrees to which these "equalised factors" influence health outcomes and what lessons can be drawn from any such observations. As pointed out by Maynard, decisions may then be made to allocate resources to those with less ability to benefit.[5] Of course, this could also involve the development of interventions which better meet the needs of such groups as opposed to interventions which do relatively well on average. This move beyond the emboldened and dotted boxes of Figure 1.1, along with its implications for systematic review, is highlighted in Chapter 10, by Birch.

Concluding comments, addressing many of the controversies and unresolved issues from Chapters 1 to 10, are provided by Drummond (Chapter 11). This is followed by a glossary of terms compiled by Currie and Manns. As this is a highly useful resource in itself, and given the work required to compile it, this glossary has been given the status of a chapter (Chapter 12).

Summary and invitation

The theoretical case for wanting to undertake economic evaluations alongside systematic reviews of effectiveness is strong. In some cases, such economic evaluations can be relatively straightforward and provide important results. We will see examples of such cases in this book. However, the conduct of such economic evaluations is not always straightforward. It will be seen that different approaches to the same underlying issue can lead to different results, that there are significant negative consequences from not using the best available evidence at the time an economic evaluation is conducted and that there is not necessarily a consensus on the best way forward. It is important that systematic reviewers thinking about conducting an economic evaluation are aware of such issues and that there may be no one best way of incorporating economics into their review process. In addition, it is necessary to think about the limitations of systematic review more generally and, also, of the limits of performing economic evaluations alongside such reviews.

Furthermore, for those more interested in the broader development of health policy, economics can make important contributions by proposing economic interventions, such as changes in incentives, which themselves require evaluation, and by analysis of factors which may be more important than interventions themselves in determining the health of the population.

If you are interested in some or all of the above, we invite you to take this journey "from effectiveness to efficiency" and enjoy *Evidence-based Health Economics*.

References

1 Egger M, Altman D, Davey-Smith G. *Systematic reviews*. London: BMJ Books, 2000.
2 Mason J, Eccles M, Freemantle N, Drummond M. A framework for incorporating cost-effectiveness in evidence based clinical practice guidelines. *Health Policy* 1999;**47**:37–52.
3 Williams A. How Archie Cochrane changed my life. *J Epidemiol Community Health* 1997;**51**:116–20.
4 Cochrane AL. *Effectiveness and efficiency: random reflections on health services*. London: Nuffield Provincial Hospitals Trust, 1972.
5 Maynard A. Evidence-based medicine: cost effectiveness and equity are ignored. *BMJ* 1996;**313**:170.
6 Evans RG, Stoddart GL. Producing health, consuming health care. *Soc Sci Med* 1990;**31**: 1347–63.
7 Drummond MF, O'Brien B, Stoddart GL, Torrance GW. *Methods for the economic evaluation of health care programmes*. Oxford: Oxford University Press, 1997.

2: Using systematic reviews in economic evaluation: the basic principles

CAM DONALDSON, MIRANDA MUGFORD,
LUKE VALE

Introduction

Accepting Cochrane's motto and, thus, the need for an economics approach to systematic review, this chapter begins by outlining the basic principles underlying economic evaluation, especially as it relates to systematic review. The remainder of the chapter returns to the practicalities of linking systematic reviews and health economics to policy questions. The possible approaches that could be taken to incorporating results from systematic reviews into economic evaluations are outlined, as well as the sources of economic data which could be used in this regard. The final section highlights the fact that economic evaluation in this context still faces some important methodological challenges.

The basics of the economic approach

In health care systems, there are never enough resources to meet all potential uses. As a result, decisions must be made about which claims will be funded, and to what levels, and which will not. The need to make choices where there is scarcity leads us to consider the economic principle of opportunity cost.

Opportunity costs express the effects of an action in terms of the forgone benefits of the next best alternative use of the set of resources used to implement that action.[1–3] If resources are used in one way, they cannot be used in other ways. Invariably, choices must be made between claims on resources each of which produces some positive outcome. As such, allocating resources to one option incurs the cost that some benefit will be lost because resources were not allocated to another option. Thus, one of the primary goals of making service delivery choices and setting health care priorities is to maximise benefits and minimise opportunity costs. To achieve this level of efficiency, information is required on both resource use (that is, costs) and benefits (that is, effectiveness) from alternative courses of action.

Randomised trials, other controlled comparisons and systematic reviews of effectiveness are methods for comparing alternative ways to treat similar groups of patients. The framework they provide is a useful vehicle for deriving and linking estimates of relative costs and effectiveness of alternative procedures, thus making it possible to determine whether a new procedure is:

- less costly and at least as effective as its comparator (ideally, the comparator is the status quo), in which case the new procedure would be judged, unequivocally, to be a better use of health care resources (in economics language, dominant and "more technically efficient"); or
- more costly, and more effective, than the comparator, in which case a judgement would have to be made about whether the extra cost of the new procedure is worth incurring given the gains in health achieved (an "allocative efficiency" question).

The allocative efficiency question brings us back to the notion of opportunity cost. Given that a new procedure is more beneficial but is going to cost more than current practice, should we allocate more resources to that area of care given the alternative uses of the resources available? For example, given that laparoscopic hernia repair is more effective than conventional surgery, should we allocate more resources to it, given that the extra cost per QALY (quality-adjusted life year) gained is £55 000,[4] and that the extra resources could be used to improve care for cancer or other needy patients?

Data on effectiveness and costs can be brought together in a matrix format (Figure 2.1) to aid in the judgement about whether a new procedure is preferable to the status quo. In Figure 2.1, it can be seen that, relative to the status quo, the new procedure could achieve (1) greater effectiveness, (2) the same level of effectiveness or (3) less effectiveness. Of course, a fourth option is possible whereby, after reviewing the literature, there is not enough evidence to make a judgement on whether the new procedure is more or less effective. Within evaluations based on randomised trials and other controlled comparisons, for example, the main aim is to identify data on the relative effectiveness of health care interventions. Systematic review, promoted most prominently by bodies such as the Cochrane Collaboration, uses techniques like meta-analysis, but also has the identification, summary and promulgation of evidence on effectiveness as its primary goal.

What economics most obviously adds to the evaluation is consideration of the resource consequences of any proposed changes in the way health care is delivered. Thus, in terms of cost, a new procedure could (A) save

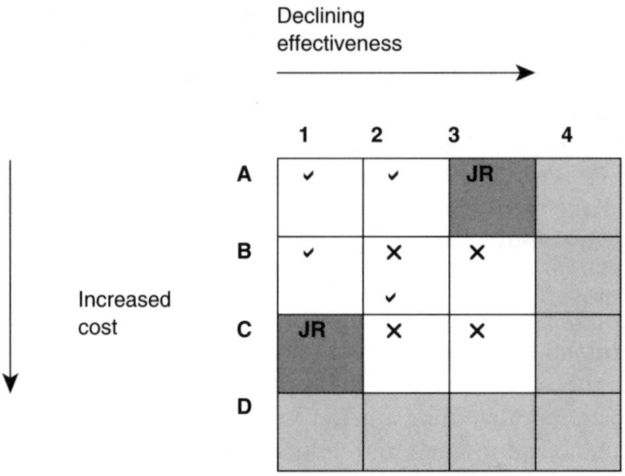

✓ = Yes/adopt ✗ = No/reject ✗ ✓ = Indifferent JR = judgement required

Effectiveness

Compared with the control treatment the experimental treatment has:

1 Evidence of greater effectiveness
2 Evidence of no difference in effectiveness
3 Evidence of less effectiveness
4 Not enough evidence of effectiveness

Cost

Compared with the control treatment the experimental treatment has:

A Evidence of cost savings
B Evidence of no difference in costs
C Evidence of greater costs
D Not enough evidence on costs

Figure 2.1 Matrix linking effectiveness with cost.

costs, (B) result in no difference in costs or (C) increase costs. (Again, there is the possibility of there being not enough evidence to judge, as represented by row D.)

Figure 2.1 is adapted from that which appeared in early editions of the Cochrane Collaboration Handbook.[5,6]* For any procedure, the optimum

* In this respect, we gratefully acknowledge other members of the Cochrane Health Economics Group: especially Ron Akehurst, Martin Buxton, Iain Chalmers, Ray Churnside, Paul Fenn, John Forbes, Alastair Gray, Jane Griffin, Sarah Howard, Tom Jefferson, Alastair McGuire, Bernie O'Brien, Andy Oxman and Adrian Towse.

position on the matrix (Figure 2.1) is square A1, where an experimental treatment would both save costs and have greater effectiveness relative to current treatment. In squares A1, A2 and B1, the new procedure is more efficient and is assigned a ✓ response to the question of whether it is to be preferred to current practice. In squares B3, C2 and C3 the new procedure is less efficient and thus receives a × response. In squares A3 and C1 a judgement would be required as to whether the more costly procedure is worthwhile in terms of the additional effectiveness gained (the allocative efficiency question again). Square B2 is neutral, as there is no difference in either costs or effectiveness. All the light grey areas in the matrix represent situations in which there is not enough evidence on effectiveness, costs or both to judge whether the new procedure is to be preferred.

Generally, cells A1, A2 and B1 (as well as B3, C2 and C3) represent three types of situation addressed by cost-effectiveness analysis (CEA). Here, CEA tells us how to achieve a given outcome at less cost or how to spend a limited amount of funds more effectively. There may be situations where effectiveness is measured in multidimensional terms, in which case a composite assessment of the value of these outcomes, in the form of quality-adjusted life years (QALYs) or healthy years equivalents (HYEs) or even willingness to pay (WTP), may be useful.

In situations represented by cells A3 and C1 the question of the additional cost of achieving the health gains becomes important. It is also useful here to have effectiveness gains valued in terms of QALYs/HYEs or willingness to pay (WTP). An incremental value of the benefits gained can then be calculated along with an incremental value of the cost incurred to achieve such a gain. Ideally, with the benefits valued in such a manner, decision makers could compare the benefits gained by the new procedure with those that would be gained by some alternative uses of the incremental resources which the new procedure would require. Thus, once again, the opportunity cost of the new procedure would be highlighted. Cost-utility and cost-benefit analyses are designed for these types of question, the former using QALYs/HYEs and the latter usually making use of monetary valuation of benefits such as WTP. (See Chapters 4 and 5 for examples of the use of WTP and QALYs, respectively.)

Thus there are two additional contributions that economic evaluation can make to systematic reviews of effectiveness. First, the matrix in Figure 2.1 shows that the economic approach adds the consideration of resource use to effectiveness evidence. By highlighting issues of technical efficiency and opportunity cost, this alone should make systematic reviews more relevant for decision making. Second, although disaggregated outcomes are of use for clinical and patient information, composite measures of the benefits of health care, in the form of QALYs, HYEs or WTP, may further aid the decision making process for resource allocation decisions. In this book, we do not go into how these economic measures of benefit (referred to as "utilities") are constructed. A certain level of knowledge is assumed and the curious reader is referred elsewhere for this[1–3] as well as to the glossary in Chapter 12. Some of the subsequent chapters use these concepts in the empirical work presented.

Putting it into practice: issues in economic evaluation and systematic review

It is important to consider whether to conduct an economic evaluation alongside a systematic review. Including economic evaluation in the review process can lead to a large increase in the workload as the amount of data that needs to be identified and abstracted increases. In addition, economic evaluation, as with many other aspects of reviewing, can be technically very challenging. For an economic evaluation, information is required on resource use, intermediate and final health outcomes and, perhaps, the strength of preferences of patients and society for health outcomes, expressed as utilities. Additionally, once these data have been obtained, they have to be combined (modelled) so estimates of efficiency can be obtained. Inclusion of an economic evaluation is likely to be worthwhile where significant amounts of health care resources are at stake and where trade-offs between costs and outcomes, or between different types of outcomes, are likely (see Box). However, once a decision is made to include economic evaluation in the review process, it is not always clear how to go about it.

Economic evaluation is important when ....

... significant amounts of health care resources are at stake; and
... where trade-offs between costs and outcomes, or between different types of outcomes, are likely.

Potential approaches for the incorporation of economics into the review

There are many alternative methods of incorporating economic evaluation into the process of systematic review. These approaches, though having the same objective, differ in their complexity and in the quality and completeness of information they require and produce. Potential approaches include:

1 Systematic review of all (economic) evaluations containing relevant data no matter what study design (for example, randomised trial,

cohort study, expert opinion) has been used to collect the baseline data (which could be referred to as the "health technology assessment approach").

2 Systematic review of effectiveness, with cost data obtained from any available economic evaluation.
3 Systematic review of effectiveness, with cost data obtained only from economic evaluations performed alongside robust study designs.
4 Systematic review of effectiveness where key "cost drivers" (the main areas where resource use differs) are identified as review outcomes which may or may not subsequently be costed by combining with relevant (local) prices.
5 Performance of a secondary economic evaluation where the systematic review of clinical effectiveness is the main source of data but secondary searches and primary data collection may be performed to identify resource use, cost and utilities.

The list of options presented above is by no means exhaustive and is illustrative of the continua of approaches that are available. Arguably, options similar to 1 and 2 above are the least compatible with the ethos of systematic review as embodied by the Cochrane Collaboration. Furthermore, comprehensive databases containing summaries of the results of economic evaluations are available or are in the process of being assembled. An example of such a database is the NHS Economic Evaluation Database, which also provides critical appraisal, funded by the Department of Health in England and produced by the NHS Centre for Reviews and Dissemination at the University of York, England (http://www.york.ac.uk/inst/crd). A further example is the Health Economic Evaluation Database (HEED) (Office of Health Economics, London).

The focus of this book will be on options 3 to 5 listed above. Whichever approach is used, each involves simplification and summing up of information about quantity and value of inputs (resources) used and outcomes experienced by patients using the alternative forms of health care under comparison. The information required for each option includes the predicted changes in: health, resource use, cost and utility. Additional factors also affect the possibility of combining evidence between studies as well as the interpretation and "transferability" of the results of an approach to other settings. These factors include:

- details of the types of care compared and the context in which they are provided;
- characteristics of the patients treated;
- how the pathways of care experienced by patients were described in terms of cost-generating events;

- the viewpoint of the analysis, which should reflect the stakeholders involved in and affected by the decision and which will affect what costs and benefits are considered; and
- the time horizon and scale of the decision to be made.

Key issues from the above list are that the quality of any given approach will be dependent upon the quality of documentation of the context of an evaluation (types of care compared and types of patients included in studies), the methods that have been used to collect and analyse the data, and the breadth of data collected (over time and across viewpoints, such as public sector only or whether patient costs are included).

The key is transparency, so that, as far as possible, results can be replicated or even altered to comply better with different local situations (for example, costs may be different in Norwich compared with not only Calgary but also Aberdeen). Thus, the context, as determined by the policy question to be addressed, will determine which studies are included, what data are collected and how the data from the studies are used. Much of this will be a matter of judgement and requires clear documentation of assumptions made. The importance of context in determining not only study design but also the design of appropriate interventions for different groups in society is addressed in greater detail later in this book, by Birch (see Chapter 10).

The following sections contain a general introduction to the types of data required for the above approaches.

Approaches primarily concerned with assembling information from reviews for use in subsequent economic evaluation

There are a number of examples of where this approach has been used.[7–10] In Chapters 3 and 4, two examples are used to demonstrate to the reader how economic evaluation can be performed alongside a systematic review and how important the economic evaluation was in making the review more relevant for decision making. The examples are protocols for the use of surfactant in the prevention and treatment of neonatal respiratory distress (Mugford) and prescribing for women prior to surgery for excision of uterine fibroids (Farquhar and Brown).

In general terms, the pieces of information required by economists in order to perform economic evaluation (based on material presented by Martin Buxton at a Cochrane Workshop in 1993) are as follows:

- identification of all main event pathways that have distinct resource implications or outcome values associated with them;
- estimation of the probabilities associated with the main event pathways, both for resource use and outcomes;

Table 2.1 Constructing a clinical event pathway for an economic evaluation.

Event pathway	Example
Clinical event	Stroke
↓	↓
Clinical event management + subsequent clinical events	Acute care and rehabilitation + sequelae and complications of treatment
↓	↓
Resources used to manage events and outcomes of events	Length of hospital stay, intensity of rehabilitation therapy, management of sequelae and complications (for example, bleeding from secondary prophylaxis) and health outcomes associated with each stage
↓	↓
Cost of resources used and utilities of outcomes	Valuation of resources using health care (and other) pay and prices and valuation of outcomes using QALYs/HYEs/WTP

- descriptive data to enable the resource consequences associated with each pathway to be measured; and
- descriptive data to enable the outcomes associated with following each pathway to be valued.

Event pathways can be used to represent different health outcomes or processes (see Table 2.1 for an example). Basically, data on two types of "outcomes" need to be collected: differences between comparison groups in terms of health outcomes (effectiveness) and differences in resource use. Guidelines regarding the collection of effectiveness and resource use data relative to each type of outcome are shown in Table 2.2 and explained below.[11]

A in Table 2.2 deals with events with important implications for health (i.e. the principal health outcomes), which should be identified. Controlled studies often report outcomes for participants up until a critical event, such as a stroke, or over a fixed time period following the intervention. With respect to economic decisions, benefits for participants after any such event are also important. Whenever possible, the distribution of these events and outcomes over time should also be recorded in order that discounting can be performed accurately.[1] There is a need for judgement about the appropriate time horizon over which to assess costs and benefits; the appropriate horizon not always being a patient's lifetime. Whenever

Table 2.2 Guidelines for collecting information for economic evaluation.

	Effectiveness	Resource use
Identification of all the main event pathways	**A** Events with important implications for health should be identified and relevant length of follow up defined. Data on health outcomes beyond clinical event (for example a stroke) should be collected if they are available	**B** Outcomes that represent resource use should be identified; especially differences in hospitalisation, when relevant. Follow up data beyond a clinical event (for example a stroke) should be collected if they are available
Estimation of probabilities associated with the main event pathways	**C** A measure of variation (for example standard deviation), as well as a point estimate (for example risk of death), should be collected if possible	**D** A measure of variation (for example standard deviation), as well as a point estimate (for example mean length of stay), should be collected if possible
Descriptive data relating to the main event pathways	**E** Data necessary to construct utilities should be collected, if required and if possible	**F** Data on resources used to manage events should be collected if they are available

possible, data reflecting important combinations of events should be collected. For example, it may be important to know whether adverse effects of a treatment occurred, and in which patients, in order for the main event pathways to be described and valued appropriately.

B in Table 2.2 deals with outcomes that represent resource use. Again, these should be identified. Outcomes that represent resource use may include any of the following: probability and length of inpatient admissions; intensity of inpatient care; probability of surgical or medical interventions or specialised care; nursing or medical staff time; medication; consumables and investigations; probability of outpatient consultation; probability of primary care consultations; day care, residential care, home services; and patient-incurred items, such as home nursing or over-the-counter drug consumption.

Resource use may be associated with initial treatment or with the consequences of treatment. For example, a stroke is a clinically important event not only in terms of outcome but also because of its resource implications. It may be important to ascertain the costs associated with care for any sequelae or complications following a stroke. Similarly, follow up data after a participant is withdrawn from a trial should be collected if possible. Data in trials being reviewed may be presented so that patients' pathways through diagnostic categories can be described. In this case, it is sometimes possible to infer costs from information about resource use in each study group.

In sum, it may be helpful for reviewers to consider explicitly which clinical outcomes included in a review are likely to have important resource implications. This can guide decisions about what, if any, data should be collected on resource use and costs associated with the main event pathways. Again, for purposes of discounting, information on the time distribution of events with resource implications is also important.[1]

C in Table 2.2 deals with measurement of effectiveness. A measure of variation, as well as a point estimate, of effectiveness should be collected if possible. There is nothing controversial in stating that data on clinical effectiveness and quality of life can and should be subjected to conventional statistical analysis. However, what is more controversial is that estimates of treatment effect can vary and this can have substantial effects on the end result of an economic evaluation. This is demonstrated in the work of Coyle and Lee (reported in Chapter 5), as well as Jefferson *et al* (Chapter 6) and Demicheli *et al* (Chapter 7).

D deals with measurement of resource use. Again, a measure of variation, as well as a point estimate, of resource use should be collected if possible. The descriptive data needed to cost an event pathway include the quantities and costs of resources used to manage events, probabilities of subsequent events, and their associated resource use and cost. In general, the types of resource use data that are most likely to be useful in subsequent economic analyses are the same as those listed above under B (outcomes that result in resource use). As the overall cost per patient is a composite, the information needed to analyse variability through statistical methods will often be lacking. Therefore, at least, the way in which any resource use information was assembled should be noted. Again, the impact on end results of variations in how cost data are compiled is explored by Coyle and Lee (Chapter 5).

E deals with valuation of health outcomes. Data necessary to construct utilities should be collected if possible. Trials may report multiple outcomes and in these circumstances, economists may wish to assess "utility". Utilities are seldom reported in trials. However, it may be possible to construct utility values from a range of measures of functional status or quality of life, and these should be reported. It should be noted that, if this is not possible, it does not mean that an economic evaluation, in which costs are considered alongside clinical outcomes without the use of utilities, cannot be done. Again, there may be variation in estimates of utilities from different sources – the impact of this variation on end results being explored (once more) by Coyle and Lee in Chapter 5.

Finally, **F** deals with valuation of resource use. Data on the costs of items of resources used to manage events should be collected if they are available. It is even less likely that a trial will have fully costed out the alternatives being compared. In this case, data on the cost of the resources used are likely to be obtained from a separate exercise, sometimes involving collaboration with a local health service accountant to obtain estimates of the unit costs of the important items of resource use.

Where money costs are presented in trials, they should be reported in reviews with caution. Financial values depend on prices, currency and time and also may be derived using a large number of sources or methods. The derivation methods, place and year should be reported with any cost variable.

Challenges in economic evaluation alongside systematic review

Guidance on quality of evidence in economic evaluations is still limited. Systematic reviews of effectiveness are formal and reproducible. No such method exists for conducting economic evaluations alongside systematic reviews.[12]

In most cases, the lengths of follow up in the trials involved in systematic reviews of effectiveness are often too short, as an economic perspective often takes a much longer-term view. Also, much of the data required for an economic evaluation may not be available from the randomised trials. In these cases, decision analytic models are often constructed in attempts to "model" the future patterns of health outcomes and resource use. Decision analysis splits the investigation into components small enough to

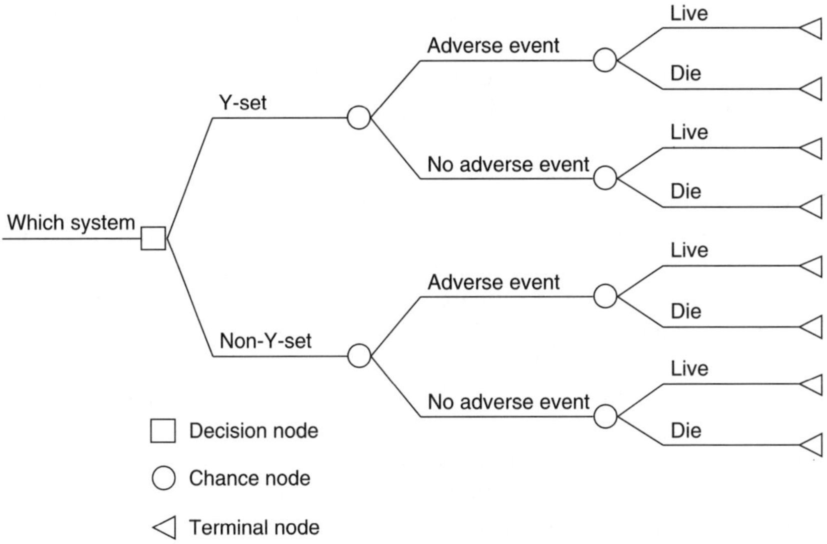

Figure 2.2 Simplified decision model for the comparison of different "connect systems" for patients on continuous ambulatory peritoneal dialysis for end stage renal disease.

be readily understood and analysed. These components are then used to model the problem's essential elements. Under this methodology, the possible chains of events (from initial choice of intervention through chance events and final outcomes) are identified in a tree structure that clearly specifies their sequence. Data are analysed by giving each possible event a valuation (either in terms of resource use, health outcome or both), and by weighting valuations for uncertain events by the probability of occurrence.

Figure 2.2 represents a simplified decision tree for the comparison of two connection systems for people with end stage renal disease who receive continuous ambulatory peritoneal dialysis (CAPD).[6] Within the model the decision is presented about whether a patient will receive CAPD with either a Y-set or non-Y-set connection system. A cost of dialysis will be incurred, the relative size of which depends on the connection system used. There is the chance that a number of adverse events may occur, such as peritonitis, access infections, switching to haemodialysis. The incidence of these adverse events as well as being a measure of effectiveness will also have cost implications as resources may be required to manage them. The cost implications per patient of treating the adverse events will be dependent upon the probability that an adverse event occurs and perhaps also its duration. In a similar way to the treatment of costs it would also be possible to use the model to estimate the patient's survival and his or her quality of life.

Problems arise in such models, where the original systematic review does not generate sufficiently long-term or disaggregated data to estimate probabilities of following specific care pathways in the decision model. Estimation of such probabilities is easier in studies based on individual patient data.

In each case of economic evaluation based on systematic review of effects of care, the model is likely to use data from other sources about the baseline risks of the key outcomes (both health and resource use). Information on resource use and cost may need to be supplemented by data from observational studies and primary data collection. This is not unusual and as was mentioned in Chapter 1 even with economic evaluation alongside a randomised trial, some of the burden of data collection (for both costs and outcomes) quite legitimately falls outwith the trial.[13] As said in Chapter 1, what is not clear, however, is which is the most appropriate source for the different types of data required (resource use, prices, patient outcomes) to conduct the evaluation. The impact of different estimates of such variables, and assessments of the quality of the outputs of economic evaluations are addressed in Chapters 5 to 8.

Conclusion

The case for wanting to undertake economic evaluations alongside systematic reviews of effectiveness is strong. What economic evaluations add to systematic reviews are (1) consideration of the resource consequences of alternative interventions under consideration and (2) methods for valuing health (and other) outcomes in a single unit such as QALYs or WTP.

Returning to the basic principles of efficiency and opportunity cost, ultimately, these pieces of information can be fed into models, such as that just outlined for the case of connection systems used in CAPD. Such models have the potential to aid policy making by determining if one connection system is more effective and less costly than the other or, if more costly as well as more effective, highlighting the magnitude of extra resources required and, therefore, the question of what the opportunity cost of these would be.

In some cases, such economic evaluations can be relatively straightforward and provide important results. Such cases will be seen in this book. However, the conduct of such economic evaluations is not always straightforward. It will be seen that different approaches to the same underlying issue can lead to different results, that there are significant negative consequences from not using the best available evidence at the time an economic evaluation is conducted and that there is not necessarily (and probably never will be) consensus on the best way forward. It is important that systematic reviewers thinking about conducting an economic evaluation are aware of such issues and that there may be no one best way of incorporating economics into their review process. It is our belief, however, that incorporation of economics into systematic review has the potential to make such reviews stronger and more relevant for decision making. The case studies in the following two chapters will illustrate precisely this.

Summary points

- Consideration of both resource use and health outcomes together enables decision makers to consider technical efficiency gains or opportunity costs from new interventions relative to current practice.
- Economic analysis can also add composite measures of the value of interventions and their outcomes, through measures such as quality-adjusted life years and willingness to pay.
- There are several different approaches to combining economic evaluations and systematic reviews of effectiveness, each will lead to different results and no one method is necessarily the best.
- For any economic evaluation, it is important to identify, measure and value costs and outcomes, and be transparent on what you did and how you did it.

References

1 Drummond MF, O'Brien B, Stoddart GL, Torrance GW. *Methods for the economic evaluation of health care programmes*. Oxford: Oxford University Press, 1997.
2 Jefferson T, Demicheli V, Mugford M. *Elementary economic evaluation in health care*. London: BMJ Books, 2nd Edition, 2000.
3 Auld C, Donaldson C, Mitton C, Shackley P. Economic evaluation. In: Detels R, Holland W, McEwan J, Omenn G, eds. *Oxford textbook of public health*. Oxford: Oxford University Press, 2001.
4 MRC Laparoscopic Groin Hernia Trial Group Writing Committee: McIntosh E, Donaldson C, Scott N, Grant A. A cost utility analysis of open versus laparoscopic groin hernia repair. *Br J Surg* 2001;**88**:653–61.
5 Cochrane Collaboration. *Cochrane Collaboration handbook*. Oxford: The Cochrane Collaboration, 1995.
6 Vale L, Donaldson C, Daly C, Campbell M, Cody J, Grant A *et al*. Evidence-based medicine and health economics: a case study of end stage renal disease. *Health Econ* 2000;**9**:337–51.
7 Mugford M, Kingston J, Chalmers I. Reducing the incidence of infection after caesarean section: implications of prophylaxis with antibiotics for hospital resources. *BMJ* 1989;**299**:1003–6.
8 Mugford M, Piercy J, Chalmers I. Cost implications of different approaches to the prevention of respiratory distress syndrome. *Arch Dis Child* 1991;**66**:757–64.
9 Smith TJ, Hillner BE. The efficacy and cost-effectiveness of adjuvant therapy of early breast cancer in premenopausal women. *J Clin Oncol* 1993;**11**:771–6.
10 Howard S, McKell D, Mugford M, Grant A. Cost-effectiveness of different approaches to perineal suturing. *Br J Midwif* 1995;**3**:587–605.

11 Akehurst R, Gray A, Buxton MJ, Chalmers I, Donaldson C *et al.* Assembling information in reviews of randomised controlled trials for subsequent cost-effectiveness analysis. Workshop Report. Oxford: UK Cochrane Centre, November 1993.
12 Mugford M. Using systematic reviews for economic evaluation. In: Egger M, Altman D, Davey-Smith G, eds. *Systematic reviews.* London: BMJ Books, 2000.
13 Drummond MF. *Economic analysis alongside controlled trials; an introduction for clinical researchers*. London: Department of Health, 1994.

3: Reviewing economic evidence alongside systematic reviews of effectiveness: example of neonatal exogenous surfactant

MIRANDA MUGFORD

Introduction

Intensive care for babies born "too soon" developed over the second half of the twentieth century. The technologies, which were costly, involved one-to-one nursing, with continuous monitoring, and life support such as giving oxygen and mechanical ventilation. In the early years of diffusion of neonatal intensive care, economic studies debated the margin of low birth weight at which costs resulting from providing neonatal intensive care outweighed the benefit,[1] and more recent studies continue to do so.[2] The high cost of neonatal intensive care technology was associated with improvements in mortality, but with diminishing effect as it was applied to more and more immature and low weight babies.

Immature lungs, which do not produce the endogenous surfactant needed within them, are particularly vulnerable to damage by mechanical ventilation. The term "respiratory distress syndrome" (RDS) is applied in diagnosis of babies who are unable to breathe without assistance. Two parallel pharmaceutical interventions were found during the 1970s that dramatically increased the ability of very preterm babies to breathe, and survive. These were, first, corticosteroids given to the mother antenatally when preterm birth was anticipated, and, second, artificial surfactant preparations administered to the baby at birth or on signs of respiratory distress. Both these technologies were adopted widely during the 1990s, and were shown to be effective in reducing neonatal mortality when compared to the intensive care treatments currently practised. Both treatments are now incorporated in clinical guidelines and used routinely in perinatal care in many places. In the UK in 2000 an episode of neonatal intensive care could be costed at anywhere between about £5000 and £150 000, and the cost of surfactant treatment is about £1000 per baby (£300–£700 per dose).

The aim of this chapter is to illustrate advantages and disadvantages of two different approaches to summing up the economic evidence about neonatal surfactant. The question of the appropriate use of surfactant is taken as the example. Should surfactant be given as soon as possible after birth in babies likely to develop RDS or should it be given only on signs of RDS?

One approach is to attempt to base an economic evaluation on the results of a systematic review of randomised controlled trials, another is synthesis based on the results of reviewing economic studies of surfactant.

A further aim of this chapter is to suggest ways in which Cochrane reviews might be adapted to provide material in a way that could be used to judge the relative economic value of the forms of care being compared. The chapter is based on the review of effectiveness of early versus delayed selective surfactant by Yost and Soll.[3]

What needs to be considered in assessing the cost-effectiveness of surfactant?

From Chapter 2, any economic evaluation needs to:

- specify the question, viewpoint (who is making the decision?) and the form of care against which the new intervention is compared;
- define the outcome(s), and the time horizon with which decision makers are concerned;
- define the types of resource use and the pathways by which resources are consumed;
- measure changes in outcomes and resource use, and apply values to these changes;
- compare the changes in costs and outcomes; and
- test variability and uncertainty.

These steps have been taken as the basis for reviewing the economic evidence.

Specifying the question: the perspective, the outcomes and time horizon

The long-term aim of neonatal care, from any perspective, is to improve the chances of healthy long-term survival for sick and immature newborn babies. In this chapter, only the short-term, health providers' perspective for the economic analysis is considered. This is partly for simplicity, but also because this is the context in which the main decisions to use surfactant have been based.

The question to be addressed here is: what is the additional cost of achieving an additional survivor at discharge from neonatal care, for babies who are at high risk of developing respiratory distress syndrome (RDS), if surfactant is given soon after birth (less than 8 hours), compared to giving surfactant later, if and when RDS is diagnosed.

Eligibility for surfactant is not simply defined, depending as it must on clinical judgement of risks at birth and subsequently. However, for the purposes of the trials that have been reported, babies were included when they met varying criteria of low gestational age, low birth weight, whether they had a chance to benefit from antenatal corticosteroid treatment, and clinical estimation of risk.

Defining outcomes of treatment for preterm babies

The objective of this economic study is modest, given the importance of longer-term outcomes both to parents and the children themselves. It does, however, maintain the simplicity of the example, which can be developed further. Even with short-term cost-effectiveness, quality of survival can also be considered. In the example taken for this chapter, measures of chronic lung problems and other major health problems in surviving babies are reported in trials and should not be lost from the economic assessment. An economic evaluation designed as a primary exercise would aim to include long-term outcomes at specified follow up points. A review of studies with the above objective would seek this information from included studies.

Defining pathways, resource use measures and costs

The pathways that might be followed by babies eligible for surfactant treatment are illustrated in Figure 3.1. Babies meeting criteria to be considered at risk may be treated with surfactant at different times. The first option (see node A in Figure 3.1) is to give surfactant at first breath to all babies who are intubated at birth, that is, prophylactically, or to give it later. This is the subject of a separate systematic review.[4] The options illustrated by node B in Figure 3.1 are those considered in this chapter and reviewed by Yost and Soll.[3]

The health care resources used in the short term by preterm babies are:

- the doses of initial treatment (surfactant); and
- care in the hospital neonatal nursery.

Costs to the health sector beyond the initial hospital stay, and to the families of the babies, are also likely to be important in studies where there

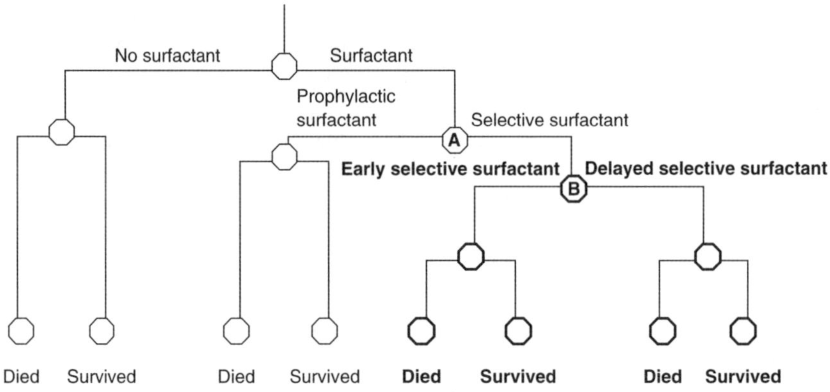

Figure 3.1 Treatment options for giving surfactant to preterm babies with high risk of respiratory distress syndrome.

are different rates of survival and hospital discharge, and relatively high levels of health problems in survivors.

Valuing changes in resource use

Advice to those conducting and reporting economic evaluations suggests that unit costs of each element of resource use should be reported separately from the quantities of health care and other resources used.[5,6] This allows readers to consider whether the costs are applicable in their own setting. If costs per patient are reported without any information on resource use, differences are more difficult to interpret. Costs reported from different times and countries need to be standardised for currency and price differences. If studies report resource use without reporting costs, then the reviewer needs to consider whether and how to seek other data about unit costs to complete the review.

Costs or outcomes occurring beyond one year from the intervention should be discounted. As the perspective of this study is less than a year, it is not likely to be a source of bias in comparing and synthesising studies.

Valuing outcomes

Although not the focus of the short-term cost-effectiveness evaluation of surfactant used in this example, similar issues arise in deriving evidence about the value of health gain measured in the studies reviewed. If utility or willingness to pay data are presented, differences in findings between studies may result from real differences in quality of life and preference, but can also be the result of methods used, patients included, or differences in underlying health states.

Variability and uncertainty

Many sources of uncertainty have been illustrated in the previous paragraphs. Differences in study design and methods, variability reported in patients treated, and assumptions needed for completion of economic analysis need to be tested in sensitivity analysis. In this case, comparison of different sources of data about costs is the focus of the chapter. In a full economic review, any aspect of the review that has known or unknown variability should be considered for its effect on the final conclusion of the economic analysis. As this is a time-consuming process, reality dictates simplification.

Sources for review of evidence for economic evaluation of surfactant

In defining the scope of the review, it was important not to exclude relevant studies, but also not to include misleading studies.

Cochrane reviews of effectiveness select studies that minimise biases in the comparison of outcomes of treatments. Although randomised trials of health interventions increasingly include economic analysis, Cochrane reviews do not generally select studies on the basis that they meet criteria for being economic evaluations, such as those defined by Drummond *et al.*[5,7] However, studies that do meet these criteria do not always qualify as trials that would be included in Cochrane reviews. This can be for a variety of reasons: some economic evaluations are based on reviews of existing trials, and some are based on effectiveness data from sources other than randomised controlled trials (RCTs).

In this chapter, findings of reviews of economic evidence from the two different "populations" of studies are compared to assess the degree to which:

- there is overlap between the reviews;
- patient allocation bias may influence the findings of economic studies; and
- relying on trials alone may miss important information about costs and outcomes.

Systematic review of randomised controlled trials of the effectiveness of early versus delayed surfactant

In their Cochrane review of early versus delayed surfactant, Yost and Soll[3] found four randomised trials meeting their criteria for the treatments compared and study design. Three trials were published in 1992 when several surfactant products were being considered for licensing in European countries[8–10] and one in 1998, with patients enrolled between October 1995 and December 1996.[11] Three trials were multicentre studies,

Table 3.1 Estimated effects of early versus delayed selective surfactant based on Cochrane review of trials.

Effect on	No. of trials reporting outcome	No. of babies	Relative risk	95% CI for relative risk Low	High	Expected rate difference (%)	NNT
Death at 28 days	4	3459	0·87	0·77	0·99	− 0·03	33
Reported mortality prior to hospital discharge	3	3039	0·90	0·79	1·01	− 0·03	33
Bronchopulmonary dysplasia (BPD)	3	3039	0·97	0·88	1·06	− 0·01	100
Chronic lung disease (CLD)	2	3007	0·70	0·55	0·88	− 0·03	33
BPD or death at 28 days	3	3039	0·94	0·88	1·00	− 0·04	25
Mortality before discharge or CLD at 36 weeks	2	3007	0·84	0·75	0·93	− 0·06	17

CI, Confidence interval; NNT, number needed to treat.
Source: Yost and Soll[3]

conducted in European centres,[8] German centres,[11] and in 229 centres in 21 countries around the world.[10] The fourth study was a single-centre trial conducted in Japan.[9]

The babies included in the trials were very preterm and/or very low weight babies who needed to be intubated within the first two hours of life. The trials all used slightly differing but overlapping categories for the inclusion criteria. The early treatment groups in all four trials included the first dose of surfactant given before the baby was two hours of age. The trials differed in how many further doses were given. Different surfactant products were used in the trials. Two trials used a synthetic surfactant[8,10] and two used natural lung extract.[9,11]

All four studies looked at neonatal mortality and three considered mortality prior to discharge from neonatal hospital care. All considered problems with oxygenation at 28 days (bronchopulmonary dysplasia, BPD) but not all used the same definition. Three trials considered the combined outcome of neonatal mortality or bronchopulmonary dysplasia. Three trials measured chronic lung disease (CLD). This measures the need for supplemental oxygen at a defined age, relating to the date the baby had been expected to be born, but is defined differently in different studies.

Table 3.1 illustrates the results of the systematic review for the main outcomes. Based on all four trials, the relative risk for neonatal mortality is 0·87 (95% CI 0·77 to 0·99). This favours the early treatment policy, but takes no account of morbidity in survivors. The relative risk for the outcome, neonatal mortality or bronchopulmonary dysplasia, based on three trials, is 0·94 (95% CI 0·88 to 1·00). This still favours the policy of giving surfactant early, but, as the confidence interval reaches 1·00, it is also possible that neither treatment is better than the other. The results for the outcome "death or chronic lung disease", based on only two trials, does favour early treatment, with a relative risk of 0·84 (95% CI 0·75 to 0·93).

The authors of the review conclude: "Early selective surfactant administration given to infants with RDS requiring assisted ventilation leads to a decreased risk of acute pulmonary injury ... and a decreased risk of neonatal mortality and chronic lung disease compared to delaying treatment of such infants until they develop established RDS." They add, under "implications for practice": "The meta-analysis would suggest that neonates with early respiratory distress should be given surfactant as early as possible."

The review by Yost and Soll[3] does not consider or comment on the economic consequences of the policy.

Review of the "economic content" of trials in the Cochrane review

The four trials included in the review were assessed as to whether they:

- included an economic evaluation;
- measured outcomes in terms of a generic measure of health gain such as life years, or quality-adjusted life years; and
- reported either costs or resource use in a way that could be used for further economic evaluation.

Economic content of the trials in the reviews of surfactant

Table 3.2 shows the number of trials known to be associated with an economic evaluation (even if reported elsewhere), and the number that presented any data about use of health care facilities (resource use) which could contribute to an economic evaluation. Table 3.2 also shows the number of reports that described the intervention and control treatments received by babies in the trial sufficient for evaluation of differences in costs of the alternative forms of care, using secondary unit cost data. Only one trial mentioned an economic evaluation, which was planned at the time of publication of the clinical results.[10] One study reported "analysis of medico-economic implications" to show "no difference between both treatment groups".[11]

Even though none of the trial reports was intended as an economic analysis, and only one of the trials was explicitly designed with economic questions in mind, it is important for reviewers not to "waste" data that might inform an economic analysis. Policies for giving surfactant might affect health care costs in the short term through the surfactant policy itself, and through its effect on the health care needs of the baby. The cost of the

Table 3.2 "Economic" content in trials of selective surfactant used early (within 2 hours of birth) versus later selective treatment of RDS.

Number of trials in Cochrane review by Yost and Soll	4
Number of trials with associated economic evaluation	1
Number of trials reporting cost differences between randomised groups	0
Number of trials reporting differences in quantities of health care resource use	2
Number of trials giving costs of intervention	0
Number of trials with any qualitative information about resource requirements for treatment of babies in trial	0
Number of trials making comment about costs	1
Number of trials making recommendations about practice	2

surfactant is determined by the size and number of doses, the profession and grade of staff and time needed for surfactant administration, and whether that person would normally be present at the place of surfactant administration. All of the surfactant trial reports described the protocol for doses and method and place of administration of surfactant. Two trials reported data about the number of doses actually given. These showed that overall use of surfactant was increased in the OSIRIS trial, from 1·65 doses in the control arm to 2·14 doses for early treatment.[10] In the German trial,[11] there was a small, but not a statistically significant, reduction in mean doses in the early treatment group.

The cost of care for the baby is reflected in length and intensity of neonatal care, and in subsequent health care contacts and readmissions after discharge. Most of the trials did include some indication of intensity of care for babies in the comparison groups, indicated by ventilator and oxygen requirements at fixed points in time (at trial entry, and at 7 and 28 days). This "snapshot" information would not allow estimation of the average number of days at each level of intensity of care for babies receiving either policy of care, until at least the point of hospital discharge, or death. Two trials did not include any continuous indicators of resource utilisation by babies in either trial allocation, although one of these collected the information for analysis in a subsequent economic study.[10] In one trial,[11] data about the mean length of stay and time in intensive care were reported in the discussion section, quoting similar data from an economic analysis based on another European study of porcine surfactant.[12]

From the trials alone, therefore, it would have been possible for the Cochrane review to comment on the economic content of the included trials, as the reports of the trials stand. Data from the trials could possibly have been extracted to model cost-effectiveness, but was not reported in the best format for this. As no unit costs are quoted in any of the trials, the reviewers would need to model the cost-effectiveness using unit costs derived from another source. In the case of Cochrane reviews, which are designed to have international applicability, it is not yet clear how this could be constructively achieved (see Chapter 5). Further, the reviewers could have commented on the papers reporting economic evaluations based on the trials included in the review. Finally, a full critical review of all the economic analyses of the economics of early versus delayed selective surfactant would have provided users of the review with the resource to investigate further the questions and methods to consider economic issues for themselves. The next section illustrates what can be found in such a review.

Systematic review of the costs and cost-effectiveness of giving surfactant

A review of the economics of neonatal care, reported in detail elsewhere,[2] included an analysis of the economics of surfactant. The search terms and strategy used for the study are reproduced as Appendix 3.1.

Petrou and Mugford[2] found that reported unit costs of neonatal care, such as *per diem* costs of intensive care, after adjustment for currency and inflation, were surprisingly similar between settings. Overall costs of neonatal care per baby differed between settings, but were predicted by the level of risk, indicated by birth weight, and prevailing mortality rates in the study. This suggests that there may be some possibility for generalisation or transfer of cost data, adjusted for currency, in economic analysis alongside reviews.

Two studies were found which investigated cost-effectiveness of early versus delayed surfactant.[12,13] A further study, not included in this review, reported the preliminary economic analysis of the OSIRIS trial.[14] Published in a journal not included in major online databases, this paper was not found in searches, and by oversight of the author (MM) was not included in the review by Petrou and Mugford. The quality of the economic studies was considered, applying the checklist suggested by Drummond *et al.*[7] No exclusions were made on the grounds of quality. A summary of the reported cost-effectiveness of early versus delayed selective surfactant is shown in Table 3.3. Unusually, all of the studies are based on effectiveness data from randomised trials or reviews of such trials. Table 3.3 illustrates that there are a range of estimates of cost-effectiveness from different, reasonably valid sources. The preliminary analysis alongside the OSIRIS trial results suggested that the early use of surfactant achieves increased survival at an additional cost well below many so-called "thresholds" for new technologies. Of course, the opportunity cost of the additional resources required would have to be considered. In sensitivity analysis, the policy of early surfactant was shown to have less good

Table 3.3 Estimates from published economic studies of cost-effectiveness of early compared to delayed selective surfactant.

Birth weight or gestational age group eligible for treatment	Study	Method for economic study	Country	Additional cost per additional survivor(£UK 1998 prices)
	Phibbs 1990[15]	Analysis of trial data	USA	Increased cost of £3110 per case and no outcome improvement
	Mugford and Howard 1993[13]	Review	Review paper	Cited Phibbs (1990)
800–1100 g	Egberts 1995[12]	Synthesis of data from reviewed studies in decision model	Netherlands	£17 773
Mean (SD) birth weight ("early" arm)	Mugford 1995[14]		International trial, UK costs	£5347
1121 (±357) g				Best scenario £1963 net cost, worst scenario higher cost associated with poorer outcome

outcomes and higher costs in the worst scenario. As this preliminary economic analysis did not use stochastic analysis of cost-effectiveness, but simple extreme scenario analysis, the likely ranges of uncertainty may have been overestimated.[16]

Follow up data from OSIRIS, the largest trial, suggested that clinical effectiveness is most marked in the first months, and that mortality after the initial hospital discharge does not change the picture.

Discussion

A review of economic studies of surfactant illustrates the range of questions that may be asked about any one health technology, and the methods that may be applied to answering them. In common with others who have also tried to sum up the results of a diverse range of economic studies on one subject,[17] the conclusion here is that this is not a very useful thing to do. One reason for this is because of the variable quality both of the design of the economic study and also of the studies from which it draws data. Economic studies will vary in their results because the question and viewpoint varies between studies, and so the variables included and the values given to them are specific to the study. However, results of studies addressing the same question from the same viewpoint have been tabulated by Petrou and Mugford,[2] and there is some consistency across costing studies in neonatal care.

A review of trials included in the Cochrane systematic reviews showed that few had reported full economic evaluations, although more had included measures of resource use. Often these measures were included as measures of clinical progress rather than to assess costs.

Currently, many Cochrane reviews do report economic outcomes that were measured within one or more trials. However, these are not usually set within a discussion of the economic issues around the technology, nor are they included in a model of the current estimated cost-effectiveness, nor is reference usually made to other studies of the economics of the technology.

This raises many questions about the limits for a Cochrane review, and about how far, by whom, how often, the review should be converted into a decision aid for economic decisions. This is the concern of health technology agencies in many countries, who are increasingly funding and using rapid reviews of cost-effectiveness evidence as a basis for decisions about funding or reimbursement priorities. Given that Cochrane reviews are seen as a vital first step in compiling these rapid reviews, the potential for Cochrane reviews at least to provide data in a more useful form for the economic analysis is obvious. This would include:

- consideration by Cochrane reviewers of the key decision points for adoption and use of the technology (and placing the review in this context);
- specification of the short- and longer-term outcomes that are likely to be of most importance for the decision to adopt the technology (to patients, funders, society and providers);
- specification of the types and nature of resource inputs likely to be consumed in this patient group, with and without the technology in question;
- assessment and reporting of cost and benefit outcomes, based on critical assessment methods for economics research, in addition to the current guidelines for judging clinical trials;
- at least cross references to economics studies of the technology, but ideally an associated critical review of the literature; and
- ideally, one or more models for cost-effectiveness or cost-utility based on the above.

This raises a great many practical and interdisciplinary problems. It is, therefore, proposed that this approach be tested by volunteer reviewers in collaboration with economists.

Summary points

- Reports of randomised controlled trials often include information relevant to economic decisions, although trialists could report such data in a more useful way for economic analysis.
- Current reporting of Cochrane reviews could be enhanced to make reviews more helpful for decision makers by including economic questions in the protocol, and reporting data about resource use, costs and economic outcomes, where necessary reporting continuous data, rather than, or in addition to, categorised outcomes.
- Full economic analyses are usually published separately from the main report of clinical trial results. A different strategy for search and critical appraisal from that used in Cochrane reviews is needed to identify and review them.

Appendix 3.1: Search strategies for economic studies of neonatal care

Free text searching

Economics: economic*, cost, costs, expenditure*;
Neonatal & care: neonat*, newborn, neonatal intensive care*, perinat*, SCBU, special care*,*low birthweight, premature*, preterm, NICU, fetus, foetus

Relevant MeSH terms

[economics (don't explode) OR economic value of life OR economics, hospital OR economics, medical OR economics, nursing OR costs and cost analysis]
and
[infant, newborn (explode, all subheadings) OR infant care (explode, all subheadings) OR nurseries, hospital OR intensive care units, neonatal OR maternal-child nursing OR perinatology OR neonatology OR fetus]

References

1 Boyle M, Torrance GW, Sinclair J. Economic evaluation of neonatal intensive care of very-low-birthweight infants. *N Engl J Med* 1983;**308**:1330–7.
2 Petrou S, Mugford M. Predicting the cost of neonatal care. In: Hansen T, McIntosh N, eds. *Current topics in neonatology IV.* London: Harcourt Health Sciences, 2000, pp. 149–74.
3 Yost CC, Soll RF. Early versus delayed selective surfactant treatment for neonatal respiratory distress syndrome (Cochrane Review). *The Cochrane Library*, Issue 3. Oxford: Update Software, 2001.

4 Soll RF, Morley CJ. Prophylactic versus selective use of surfactant for preventing morbidity and mortality in preterm infants (Cochrane Review). *The Cochrane Library*, Issue 3. Oxford: Update Software, 2001.
5 Drummond MF, O'Brien B, Stoddart GL, Torrance GW. *Methods for the economic evaluation of health care programmes*. Oxford: Oxford University Press, 1997.
6 Evers SM, Van Wijk AS, Ament AJ. Economic evaluation of mental health care interventions. A review. *Health Econ* 1997;**6**:161–77.
7 Drummond M, Jefferson T. Guidelines for authors and peer reviewers of economic submissions to the BMJ. The BMJ Economic Evaluation Working Party. *BMJ* 1996;**313**:275–83.
8 The European Exosurf Study Group. Early or selective surfactant (colfosceril palmitate, Exosurf) for intubated babies at 26 to 29 weeks' gestation: a European double blind trial with sequential analysis. *Online Journal of Current Clinical Trials* 1992;doc no. 28.
9 Konishi M, Fujiwara T, Chida S, Maeta H, Shimada S, Kasai T *et al.* A prospective randomised trial of early versus late administration of a single dose of surfactant-TA. *Early Hum Devel* 1992;**29**:282.
10 The OSIRIS Collaborative Group. Early versus delayed neonatal administration of a synthetic surfactant – the judgement of OSIRIS. *Lancet* 1992;**340**:1363–9.
11 Gortner L, Wauer R. Early versus late surfactant treatment in preterm infants of 27 to 32 weeks' gestational age. A multicenter controlled clinical trial. *Pediatrics* 1998; **102**:1160.
12 Egberts J. Theoretical changes in neonatal hospitalisation costs after the introduction of porcine-derived lung surfactant ('Curosurf'). *Pharmacoeconomics* 1995;**8**:324–42.
13 Mugford M, Howard S. Cost-effectiveness of surfactant replacement in preterm babies. *Pharmacoeconomics* 1993;**3**:362–73.
14 Mugford M. Cost-effectiveness of policies for surfactant use based on the results of the OSIRIS trial: a preliminary analysis. *Neonatal Monitor* 1995;**12**:10–12.
15 Phibbs CS, Phibbs RH, Tooley WH *et al.* The cost-effectiveness of synthetic therapy for neonatal respiratory distress syndrome. *Clinical Research* 1990;**38**:178a [conference abstract].
16 Briggs AH, Gray A. Handling uncertainty in economic evaluation of healthcare interventions. *BMJ* 1999;**319**:635–8.
17 Jefferson T, Demicheli V, Rivetti D, Deeks J. Cochrane reviews and systematic reviews of economic evaluations. *Pharmacoeconomics* 1999;**16**:85–9.

4: The place of economic analyses in systematic reviews: a clinician's viewpoint

CINDY FARQUHAR, PAUL BROWN

Introduction

Clinical decision making has traditionally involved listening to patients, arranging appropriate tests, reaching a diagnosis, considering options for treatment and then making a decision. Clinicians are trained to offer patients the very best available treatments. Unfortunately, the information on which to base the decision is often incomplete, does not always consider the risks and lacks the perspective of both those who fund health care and of the patient.

To illustrate this approach, consider the following scenario: a 33-year-old woman with two children consults a gynaecologist with heavy menstrual bleeding and is found to have large uterine fibroids. The gynaecologist suggests two alternative surgical procedures – a hysterectomy (removal of the uterus and cervix) or a myomectomy (where the uterus is conserved and just the fibroids are removed). Her fibroids are too large to be removed without a large vertical midline incision. The woman is concerned that the surgery will be disfiguring and asks about alternative surgical procedures. The gynaecologist is aware of studies showing that a three month treatment of gonadotrophin releasing hormone agonists (GnRHa) will reduce the size of fibroids and allow for better surgical outcomes (a transverse incision for a myomectomy or a vaginal route for a hysterectomy – both more cosmetically appealing). However, the treatment may have some adverse effects and is costly. The gynaecologist wonders whether the benefits to the woman from the treatment are likely to outweigh the adverse effects and the cost. The gynaecologist considers asking whether the patient would be prepared to pay for the GnRHa treatment, knowing that it is not funded in the public health system (or under some managed care arrangements). Thus, the gynaecologist is left to consider whether the resources needed for this procedure would be better spent on other health interventions.

Clinicians often face situations where there is information demonstrating the benefits from an intervention or treatment, but little context in which to understand how much their patients will value these benefits and whether the benefits are significant enough to merit expending scarce resources. The value of providing the intervention can only be judged when benefits, harms and costs are all considered. The purpose of this chapter is to highlight how economic evaluations can assist clinicians in making these decisions. Specifically, the chapter describes how evidence from a systematic review can be used in an economic evaluation, how the total cost of treatment (including the long-term costs) can be estimated, how to combine the benefit and cost information in meaningful ways, and a possible method of identifying whether the benefits are worth the cost.

Clinical and economic issues

Uterine fibroids are a commonly occurring benign tumour of the uterus in women of reproductive age. They occur in one in four women over the age of 36 years and are the most common cause of major surgery in premenopausal women.[1–3] Fibroids (also known as myoma) may occur throughout any part of the uterus. The most troublesome fibroids are those that enlarge the uterine cavity, namely intramural and submucous fibroids. Although fibroids may occur at any time before the menopause, they are most commonly seen in women in their 30s or 40s. As fibroids are oestrogen dependent they decrease in size after the menopause. During pregnancy, fibroids may enlarge and occasionally undergo a painful degeneration. They may interfere with conception and they are associated with heavy menstrual bleeding.

Two operative procedures are available to women with uterine fibroids. A *hysterectomy* (removal of the uterus and cervix) is typically performed when a woman has heavy menstrual bleeding and has completed childbearing. The procedure can be performed via an abdominal or vaginal approach. The vaginal approach is typically preferred, as abdominal wounds are considered more unsightly and are associated with higher complication rates.[4] When surgery is performed abdominally, however, the preferred method is to use a transverse rather than a vertical incision in order to minimise scarring, and to reduce pain and infection.

An alternative procedure is a *myomectomy* in which the fibroid is removed but the uterine muscle and endometrium are left intact. As with a hysterectomy, the incision can be either transverse or vertical. This procedure is preferred for women of childbearing age since, unlike the hysterectomy, the myomectomy preserves the chance of the woman remaining fertile. However, myomectomies are associated with an increased risk of haemorrhage and infection from the operation. Furthermore, a significant number of women have a recurrence of fibroids within five years of the procedure, with a hysterectomy being an option at that point.[3,5] Hysterectomy is more frequently undertaken than myomectomy.

As fibroids are oestrogen dependent, medication that lowers oestrogen levels may be effective in arresting the growth of fibroids. Past attempts to treat fibroids with progestogenic agents (such as medroxyprogesterone acetate) were unsuccessful due to the difficulty of obtaining sufficient reductions in oestrogen levels. However, the introduction of gonadotrophin (GnRHa) analogues allows reductions in oestrogen levels comparable to the range after menopause.

Evidence of effectiveness of treatment

Previous studies have demonstrated that GnRHa treatment can result in fibroid shrinkage of 30–60%.[3,6,7] Several factors preclude GnRHa treatment as a permanent solution, including the need for continuous treatment (fibroids will return to their original size once treatment ceases), the high cost of the drug (approximately NZ$400 per month) and adverse effects associated with low oestrogen levels (for example, hot flushes and vaginal dryness). However, GnRHa has been suggested as a preoperative treatment prior to hysterectomy and myomectomy and a systematic review of 21 randomised controlled trials has reported that preoperative treatment with GnRHa can lead to statistically significant clinical benefits.[5] In the study presented here the results describe the cost per abdominal entry avoided (for hysterectomies) and cost per vertical incision avoided (when an abdominal incision is necessary). The use of preoperative GnRHa for hysteroscopic or laparoscopic surgery was not considered in this study as no randomised controlled trials of preoperative GnRHa in association with those procedures were found.

The primary benefit from GnRHa treatment is the increased probability of having a preferred surgical outcome.

First, when a hysterectomy is performed, treatment with GnRHa increases the likelihood of having a vaginal rather than abdominal approach from 12% to 38% (odds ratio (OR) 4·7, 95% CI 3·0–7·4) and when an abdominal approach is used, treatment with GnRHa increases the probability of a transverse rather than a vertical incision from 67% without the treatment to 84% with the treatment (OR 2·8, 95% CI 1·8–4·3). Other outcomes are a decrease in blood loss (58 ml), shorter operating time (six minutes) and shorter length of stay (one day).

Second, for those undergoing myomectomy, all women receiving the GnRHa treatment were able to have a transverse incision (compared with only 67% for those without the treatment) (OR 8·95, 95% CI 1·3–60·1). However, the treatment increases the likelihood of a recurrence of fibroids. Whereas only 28% of the women might expect a recurrence after

Table 4.1 Probabilities of outcomes with hysterectomy and myomectomy with and without GnRHa.

			No treatment (%)	Treatment with GnRHa (%)
Hysterectomy	Vaginal approach		12	38
	Abdominal	transverse	59	52
		vertical	29	10
Myomectomy	Abdominal	transverse	67	100
		vertical	33	0
	Recurrence		28	65

Source: Matta *et al*[6]

treatment, 65% of those receiving GnRHa might expect a recurrence (OR 4·0, 95% CI 1·1–14·7). Other outcomes are a decrease in the blood loss during surgery (67 ml), and that the potential for pregnancy is maintained. There was no difference in the length of stay. The resulting final probabilities are shown in Table 4.1 and in Figure 4.1.

The systematic review of evidence reduces the uncertainty about outcomes that can result when studies are considered individually. On the strength of this information, it would seem that women treated with GnRHa can expect an increased likelihood of a preferred surgical outcome. There are few adverse effects directly from the treatment (or at least little available information), although women having a myomectomy will have an increased likelihood of a recurrence of fibroids.

Presenting the benefits

Having identified the types of benefits that are likely to result, the next step is to express the benefits in a meaningful way. The main benefits, as well as potential adverse effects, are presented in Table 4.2. For a hysterectomy, the existence of three possible surgical outcomes (a vaginal incision, transverse incision or vertical incision) presents a challenge. The results seem to suggest that while treatment increases the chance of the preferred outcome (vaginal) and decreases the chance of the least preferred (vertical), it reduces the likelihood of the middle option (transverse incision). This creates a problem in expressing the results, namely how to weigh the increased likelihood of a preferred outcome against the decreased likelihood of a next preferred option.

One way around this problem is to express the outcomes as only a choice of alternatives, but in two ways. Given that the outcomes can be ranked in preference, it is possible to express the benefits from treatment as increasing the likelihood of the preferred alternative relative to all others

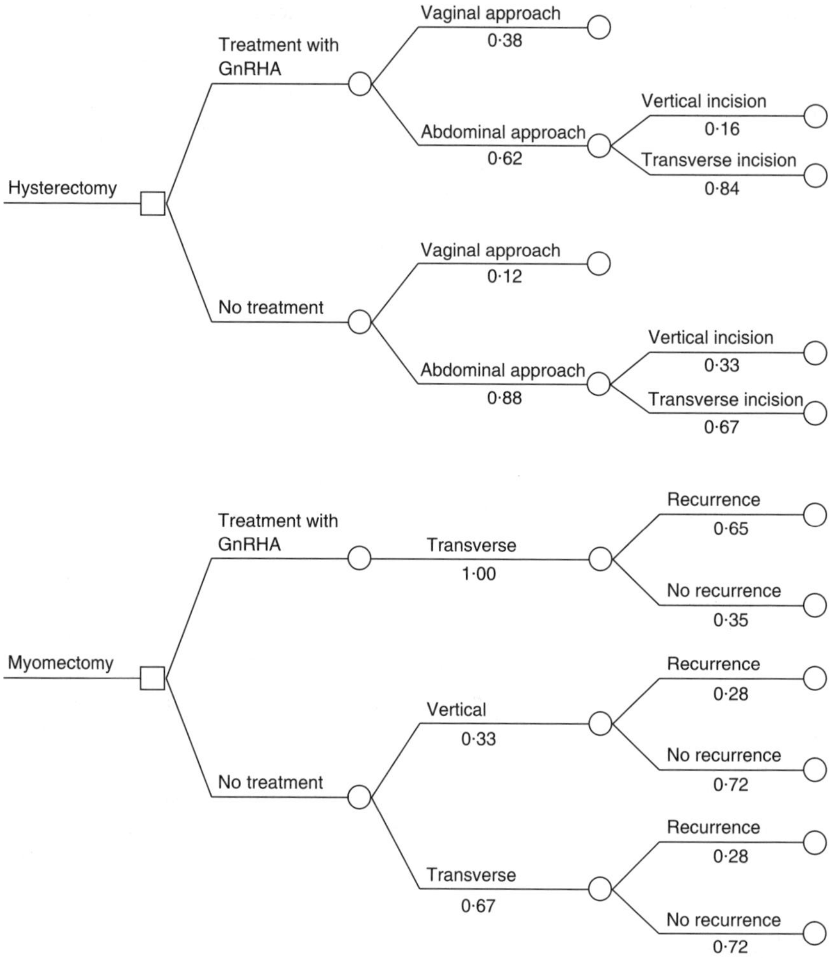

Figure 4.1 Probabilities associated with treatment.

(from 12% to 28%) and as decreasing the likelihood of the least preferred alternative (from 29% to 10%).

This problem does not exist for myomectomies as the primary benefit from treatment is the increased likelihood of having a transverse incision (from 67% to 100%). However, myomectomies pose another problem: treatment increases the risk of a recurrence of fibroids. These women are likely to require a hysterectomy within two years. Thus, the challenge is how to factor this aspect into the analysis.

One way to include the consequences of a recurrence is to factor in the increased likelihood of a hysterectomy. There is little information available on the percentage of recurrences that result in a hysterectomy. This leads

Table 4.2 Summary of treatment effects with GnRHa.

	Primary benefit	Secondary benefits	Adverse events
Hysterectomy	Increased vaginal hysterectomy	Decreased blood loss Shorter surgical time Shorter length of stay	Hot flushes Headaches Additional consultations
	Increased transverse incisions	No abdominal wound (vaginal hyst. only) Decreased pain Reduced complications	Delay in surgery (3 months) Pain of injections or insertions
Myomectomy	Increased transverse incisions	Decreased blood loss Shorter surgical time Shorter length of stay Decreased pain Reduced complications	Hot flushes Headaches Additional consultations Increased likelihood of recurrence Delay in surgery (3 months) Pain of injections or insertions

to an additional cost (as shown in the analysis below). But there is also the loss women feel from having a hysterectomy at some point in the future. Unfortunately, the systematic review provides little information on the extent women having a myomectomy would want to avoid having a hysterectomy. Thus, while it is straightforward to include the cost of recurrence to the medical system in the economic analysis, the systematic reviews offer little evidence on the intangible adverse consequences and, thus, the gains from avoiding them.

Cost of preoperative GnRHa

Having identified the benefits from the treatment (increased probability of a preferred surgical outcome), the next step is to estimate the cost associated with treatment and with no treatment. There are a number of issues to decide when estimating costs, such as the types of costs to include (direct, indirect and/or intangibles), the length of time over which to observe costs and whether to discount costs in the future. In this present study, the costs of medical care to both the health system (for example, consultation, treatment and hospitalisation) and to the patient (lost wages due to treatment) were considered. However, no evidence was available about the other types of costs (such as cost to caregivers and other medical expenses).

Costs associated with three stages of the treatment were examined: preoperative phase (commencing three months before surgery), the intraoperative phase and the postoperative period (three months). Thus, the time period for the study was six months. Only direct costs to the health sector and to the patients were examined. The health care resources used are summarised in Table 4.3.

Table 4.3 Health care resource usage.

	Preoperative phase	Intraoperative phase	Postoperative phase
Hysterectomy			
Treatment with GnRHa	3 consultations for treatment plus 10% chance of additional consultation	Surgery: 54 minutes Hospital stay: 2 days for vaginal approach, 4 days for an abdominal approach	1 consultation
No treatment		Surgery: 60 minutes Hospital stay: 2 days for a vaginal approach, 4 days for an abdominal approach	1 consultation
Myomectomy			
Treatment with GnRHa	3 consultations for treatment plus 10% chance of additional consultation	Surgery: 54 minutes Hospital stay: 3 days	1 consultation plus 65% chance of reoccurrence
No treatment		Surgery: 60 minutes Hospital stay: 4 days	1 counsultation plus 28% chance of reoccurrence

Preoperative phase

Treatment includes monthly doses of GnRHa analogue. This medication is not subsidised in New Zealand. The price used in the analysis was the market (unsubsidised) price.

To administer treatment, three injections were required (at one month intervals). Injections were administered at a gynaecology outpatient clinic. Previous studies indicate that approximately 10% of the women will require a consultation due to adverse effects from the medication.[5] The cost of the consultation is included. The average time needed for a consultation is assumed to be one hour (including travel time). Value of time from work was assessed using the average hourly wage rate for women in New Zealand.[8]

Hospitalisation phase

As mentioned above, the cost savings of GnRHa treatment result from a lower risk of complications from surgery and post-surgical infections. These savings are reflected in shorter surgery time and a shortened hospital stay.

Total theatre costs for surgery were determined using the average cost per minute of theatre time and the number of minutes per surgery. The cost assumes the theatre team consists of a consultant gynaecologist, a consultant anaesthetist and three surgical nurses. Average theatre time was available from the systematic review. The average cost per minute is based on the market rate charged by the National Women's Hospital, Auckland to private patients. As such, it includes both variable (staff and supplies) and fixed (overhead) costs associated with running the hospital.

The participant's stay in the hospital was costed using the number of days in each ward (for example, intensive care and general medical) and the average cost per day in the general medical ward. As with the theatre cost, ward cost per day uses market prices charged by the National Women's Hospital to private patients. Note that the cost per ward day includes normal use of resources (such as nurse time and standard medication). Because the hospital includes the use of antibiotics in these estimates, it is not necessary to cost the price of adverse events and infections separately. The additional cost will be reflected in the increased hospital stay (although not the pain and suffering incurred by the patient). The systematic review also indicated that treatment with GnRHa analogues did result in less blood loss and pre-and postoperative haemoglobin. However, although the difference was statistically significant, the reductions (58 ml – one unit of blood is 500 ml) were neither clinically nor economically significant. Overall, blood transfusions were not significantly reduced.

Postoperative phase

One routine consultation at two to three months after surgery was priced at the market rate. One hour's lost wages was used for the patient's time.

As discussed above, some women receiving a myomectomy will redevelop fibroids after surgery. The evidence suggests that a significant number of women who have a recurrence of fibroids receive a hysterectomy.[5,9] As no evidence is available on the relative probabilities of each outcome, the subsequent analysis will assume that 50% of all recurrences result in a hysterectomy within two years after surgery, with the cost of the hysterectomy included as an additional cost (with the rest receiving no additional treatment). It is assumed these women will have the hysterectomy an average of two years after surgery. This long-term cost will be discounted at an annual rate of 6%.[10]

Monetary valuation of costs

Having identified the resources used, the next step is to apply unit costs to each item. In the current study, either market prices were used (such as price per GP consultation) or prices obtained from hospitals (for example, cost of surgery per minute). These are described in Table 4.4. Arriving at a final price requires consideration of both the amount of resources required and the probability of those resources being used. For instance, given that there was a 10% chance of having a GP visit due to adverse effects, the expected price per patient for adverse effects was the cost of the consultation times the appropriate probability. The final costs are shown in Table 4.5.

Table 4.4 Cost estimates for all aspects of care (NZ$).

	Unit	Unit cost	Alternative values used during sensitivity analysis
Preoperative			
GnRHa	Per treatment	370	High: 555 Low: 185
GnRHa treatment	Per consultation	120	High: 180 Low: 60
Patient time off work for treatment	Hourly wage rate	20	Wages and time off work: High: 30 @ 3 hr Low: 10 @ 1 hr
Extra consultation for side effects	Per consultation	120	Consultation High: 180 Low: 60
Time off work	Hourly wage rate	20	Wages and time off work: High: 30 @ 3 hr Low: 10 @ 1 hr
Hospitalisation phase			
Theatre costs	Per minute	20	High: 30 per min Low: 10 per min
Length of stay	Per day	450	High: 600 per day Low: 300 per day
Postoperative phase			
Consultation	Per consultation	120	High: 180 Low: 60
Time off work	Hourly wage rate	20	Wages and time off work: High: 30 @ 3 hr Low: 10 @ 1 hr

NZ$ = New Zealand dollars at 2000 prices.

Economic evaluation

The results from the analysis are summarised in Table 4.6. Columns 1 and 2 show the cost per outcome. That is, it costs approximately NZ$1190 per patient in order to obtain an increase of 26% in the probability of having a vaginal rather than an abdominal hysterectomy, NZ$1190 in order to have an increase of 19% in the probability of avoiding a vertical hysterectomy, and NZ$1535 in order to have an increase of 33% in the probability of avoiding a vertical myomectomy. The last column translates these numbers into an expected cost of one additional patient receiving the desired outcome. For instance, the cost that can be expected for one person to receive a vaginal rather than an abdominal hysterectomy is NZ$4577.

Table 4.5 Analysis of costs for hysterectomy and myomectomy (NZ$).

		Treatment with GnRHa		No treatment	
		Units	Cost	Units	Cost
Hysterectomy					
Preoperative	GnRHa	3 @ 370	1110		
		3 @ 120			
	Consultation	3 @ 20	420		
	Additional consultation	10% of 1 @ 120 and 1 @ 20	14		
Hospitalisation	Surgical time (min)	54 @ 20	1080	60 @ 20	1200
	Length of stay:				
	Vaginal approach	38% of 2 @ 450	342	12% of 2 @ 450	108
	Abdominal (transverse or vertical)	62% of 4 @ 450	1116	88% of 4 @ 450	1584
Postoperative	Consultation	1 @ 120	120	1 @ 120	120
		1 @ 20	20	1 @ 20	20
Total cost			**4222**		**3032**
Myomectomy					
Preoperative	GnRHa	3 @ 370	1110		
		3 @ 120			
	Consultation	3 @ 20	420		
	Additional consultation	10% of 1 @ 120 and 1 @ 20	14		
Intraoperative	Surgical time (min)	54 @ 20	1080	60 @ 20	1200
	Length of stay (days)	3 @ 450	1350	4 @ 450	1800
Postoperative	Consultation	1 @ 120	120	1 @ 120	120
		1 @ 20	20	1 @ 20	20
Cost of reoccurence	Hysterectomy	50%*65% of $3032/(1\cdot06)^2$	985	50%*28% of $3032/(1\cdot06)^2$	424
Total cost			**5099**		**3564**

NZ$ = New Zealand dollars at 2000 prices.

Table 4.6 Cost-effectiveness of treatment with GnRHa.

	Cost difference per patient (NZ$)	Increased probability per patient (%)	Cost for one additional patient to receive the desired outcome (NZ$)
Hysterectomy			
Vaginal rather than abdominal approach	4222 −3032	38 −12	1190/0·26 =
	1190	26	4577
Avoiding a vertical incision	1190	29 −10	1190/0·19 =
		19	6263
Myomectomy			
Avoiding a vertical incision	5099 −3564	100 −67	2096/0·33 =
	1535	33	4651

NZ$ = New Zealand dollars at 2000 prices.

Valuing the differences

The results shown in Table 4.6 present the cost of obtaining an increase in desired outcomes. Left unanswered, however, is whether these benefits are worth the expense. We are in cell C1 of the matrix presented in Chapter 2. In order to make this determination, the clinician and patient must make a judgement on the value of these increased benefits.

One type of evidence to consider when making this determination is the value women place on the relevant outcomes. Unfortunately, the systematic review provided no evidence on the value women place on these outcomes.[5] Specifically, there is no indication of the value women place on the decreased hospital stay, the reduced pain and suffering during recovery, the impact of adverse effects experienced either as a result of taking the medication, or how much women value the reduced scarring associated with a vaginal approach (hysterectomy) or a transverse incision (hysterectomy and myomectomy). The question of whether or not the treatment is worth it is not established by the studies or the basic economic evaluation.

One method used by economists to establish the value that women place on the different outcomes is a contingent valuation survey in which women are asked to express the maximum amount they would be willing to pay to avoid or obtain certain outcomes. For the present study, 30 women in New Zealand were asked their willingness to pay for the various treatment options.* After reading the description of the likely effects of treatment and the expected outcomes, women were asked what was the maximum they would be willing to pay to have (a) a vaginal over an abdominal approach, (b) a transverse rather than a vertical incision (should an abdominal approach be required) and (c) a myomectomy instead of a hysterectomy. Other reports have used this approach in order to gain an idea of how women value the benefits of medical care.[11,12] Although this evidence is not a substitute for a thorough examination of quality of life differences, it does provide a rough estimate of the amount women value the various outcomes.

When asked to imagine they were to have a hysterectomy, 83% (26 of 30) of the women indicated that they would prefer a vaginal to an abdominal approach. Of those 83%, the average amount they were willing to pay was NZ$644 for a vaginal hysterectomy (ranging from 200 to 2000). (In the study, it was assumed that women generally prefer treatments that are less cosmetically scarring. Therefore, preferences for the abdominal approach are assumed to result from not fully understanding the implications of the surgery – thus highlighting a potential problem of the willingness to pay approach. As will be seen below, similar assumptions were made with respect to other choices within the questionnaire.) When asked to choose between a transverse and vertical incision for abdominal hysterectomy, 93% chose the former. The average willingness to pay for this outcome was NZ$594 (ranging again from 200 to 2000).

These estimates are similar to the average responses by women when asked to imagine they were to have a myomectomy. Ninety per cent (27 of 30) indicated that they would prefer a transverse incision and were willing to pay an average of NZ$792 for that outcome (ranging from 200 to 2000) (see Table 4.7).

As mentioned above, one limitation of GnRHa preoperative treatment for myomectomy was the increased risk of recurrence. Assuming that the recurrence leads to a 50% chance of a hysterectomy within two years, then the treatment is associated with the loss of possible fertility for a significant portion of the women. As an indication of the value women place on retaining the possibility of remaining fertile, the women were asked to indicate their willingness to pay for having a myomectomy rather than a hysterectomy. Of the 73% (11 of 15 respondents) who preferred a myomectomy, their average willingness to pay was NZ$4150 (ranging from 300 to 15 000). Thus, factoring the possibility of needing a hysterectomy in the future, the overall willingness to pay for treatment for women having a myomectomy was only NZ$25.

* The women were recruited at random from the general public. The average age and household income of the respondents was 38·3 years and approximately NZ$68 000 respectively. All resided in Auckland, New Zealand.

Table 4.7 Comparing cost of treatment with willingness to pay (NZ$).

	Average from willingness to pay questionnaire (SD)	Expected cost of treatment[a]
Hysterectomy		
Vaginal rather than abdominal approach	644 (447)	4577
Avoiding a vertical incision	594 (407)	6263
Myomectomy		
Avoding a vertical incision	792 (516)	
Avoding a hysterectomy	4150 (5016)	
Net willingness to pay to avoid a vertical incision	792– 0·5* (0·65–0·28)* 4150 = 25†[b]	4651

NZ$ = New Zealand dollars at 2000 prices.
[a] From Table 4.4.
[b] The figure of NZ$25 comes from 792 (the WTP for treatment) minus [the net increased probability of a recurrence within two years (0·65–0·28) multiplied by the probability of needing a hysterectomy (0·5) multiplied by the estimated welfare loss of 4150 in the event of a hysterectomy].

A final note on the willingness to pay study is that the method has been used simply to illustrate the potential of the approach. The study could have been done differently; for example, by asking women to assume they will have a hysterectomy and then asking them about their willingness to pay for the drugs, incorporating all future effects the drug would have on increasing probabilities of preferred outcomes, all in one scenario. The same could have been done for myomectomy. Of course, this task would have been more demanding of respondents.

Conclusions on preoperative GnRHa treatment

This economic evaluation aimed to assess the costs of avoiding vertical incisions or an abdominal approach for hysterectomy using outcome data from a systematic review of 26 trials from a number of different settings (all appropriately in gynaecological surgery) and a number of different countries.[5] This approach should increase the likelihood that the outcomes are valid and accurate. It is also acknowledged that in everyday practice the outcomes are unlikely to be as good as the clinical trials and therefore any of the benefits may be actually less than stated.

Although there were some significant clinical differences (operating time, blood loss, anaemia), these were of little consequence either clinically or economically. The only outcomes that were of clinical importance were avoided abdominal surgery (increased vaginal hysterectomy) and a reduction in vertical incisions (an increase in transverse incisions), and in the case of hysterectomy, one less day in hospital. Overall, the cost to the government of one avoided abdominal surgery or avoided vertical incision was considerable. For example, the cost of one hysterectomy is approximately NZ$4500, whereas the cost of avoiding an incision is similar and the cost of avoiding a vertical incision is greater. The monetary estimates of benefit from the willingness to pay survey provided some information on the value women place on the benefits. It was considerably lower than the cost of one avoided surgical procedure. Therefore, although it is unlikely that preoperative GnRHa analogues for women with uterine fibroids would be funded by third party payers such as insurers or government, there may be some women who are prepared to pay.

This case study sought to describe the added value of including an economic analysis for clinicians making treatment decisions. There are a number of "drivers" that influence clinical decision making – patients' preferences, financial incentives that may accompany one treatment option and educational inputs. In the case presented in this chapter, many clinicians have received convincing educational and promotional material about the statistically significant improvements that result from shrinking fibroids prior to hysterectomy and myomectomy. However, when this is fully analysed from an economic point of view the benefits accrued are small and do not appear to justify the cost. Qualifications of this statement, however, are that more work is needed to test the robustness of this conclusion by use of sensitivity analysis and that more detailed work on patient preferences is required. Furthermore, unit costs and preferences may differ across different contexts.

Discussion

Systematic reviews are now considered one of the best sources of evidence about health care interventions. The systematic review methodology, where data from more than one study are combined, means that an increased sample size results and furthermore that the information is likely to be able to be applied across more than one setting. For example, only two of the eight studies of antenatal corticosteroids in the prevention of death from respiratory distress syndrome of the preterm newborn infant demonstrated benefit, but the result of the meta-analysis showed a 50% reduction in risk of death.[13] A further example is the meta-analysis of studies of critically ill patients which demonstrated increased deaths amongst those receiving albumin although few of the 34 individual studies demonstrated this harm.[14] However, problems arise where the evidence is mixed or where there are benefits but the treatment is costly, or where valuing the benefits is difficult.

Economic analysis alongside systematic reviews can provide a way of addressing these issues. In particular, the use of economic data has the potential to allow clinicians to see whether or not statistically significant improvements in clinical outcomes are worthwhile applying in the clinical setting. It provides additional information and helps put the effectiveness data into perspective. Some improvements may become meaningless when combined with large cost differences associated with one option or the other.

How are clinicians to use this economic information? How should these findings be interpreted? Why should clinicians care about costs? The basic economic evaluation in this chapter demonstrated the cost per case avoided. The economic viewpoint is to consider the "opportunity costs". That is, if this money was not spent on this intervention where might it be better spent? In this case study, for every vertical incision avoided one or two additional hysterectomies could be undertaken. As a clinician, the additional cost did not appear to justify the benefits of avoiding certain surgical outcomes and therefore the value that women place on the outcomes was sought by conducting a willingness to pay survey. However, there are a number of limitations of the willingness to pay survey. It is possible that women did not understand the questions and that women actually facing surgery in the near future would respond differently. In the end, the willingness to pay information is only useful with the other economic information. The overwhelming impression from the combination of the cost and effectiveness data and the information from the willingness to pay survey is that there are few convincing reasons for clinicians to use this treatment in the future. However, once again, the reader should be reminded of the qualifications at the end of the previous section. Furthermore, the willingness to pay work undertaken elicited values for certain surgical outcomes and multiplied them by the probability of those outcomes occurring. An alternative approach would incorporate such probabilities into the descriptions given to respondents and, thus, directly into the valuations.

What are the barriers that may potentially affect clinicians taking cost into clinical decision making? It is likely that the different health care systems that clinicians work in will affect their acceptance of economic data. Another barrier may be the culture that many health care professionals have been trained and are accustomed to practise in. For example, many doctors work independently and do not appreciate having decisions being influenced by external pressures such as cost. Considering cost in the decision making process is a relatively new phenomenon and some clinicians may continue to ignore cost information believing that the more expensive options must be better and will result in improved health outcomes. This is certainly often the case in choosing between different pharmaceuticals and in making decisions about screening. There may also be some resistance from doctors to this approach because of the failure of evidence from systematic reviews to take individuals and subgroups into account. The averaging effect of the statistical analyses of clinical trials and systematic reviews means that there is a tendency to treat all patients as if they were "average" or will have an "average response" to treatment (see Chapter 10 for a more detailed discussion of this issue). It is often felt that there is little place to accommodate variability in either clinical outcomes or patients' preferences within the evidence-based medicine model. This is obviously a problem to doctors who have been trained to deal with patients individually. How to combine the two approaches is a challenge for clinicians who wish to be evidence-based but also wish to treat each patient on a case-by-case basis.

Few health care professionals have had exposure to health economic evaluations of care let alone a discussion of the appropriateness of the different approaches. Many health care providers view economic analyses with a certain degree of scepticism. Is this just another attempt to limit health care spending by those who fund health care? Is this an attempt to encourage the uptake of certain options over others? The concepts of "allocative efficiency" and "opportunity costs" should be considered as an important input to good medical decision making whether it is for new clinical guideline recommendations or for individual patient care. Yet, few clinicians understand these concepts and it is not uncommon for various economic terms to be confused or misused. There is a need for medical education, particularly at a postgraduate level, to consider teaching these concepts. After all, most individuals apply these approaches to their personal finances and it should not be difficult to extrapolate them to medical decision making. Over the past decade there has been a steady rise in health economics within clinical topics and an increase in the number of guidelines that now include clinical cost-effectiveness.[15,16] Furthermore, it could be argued that it is an ethical responsibility to consider these issues as the savings on spending could be directed to other areas of health with greater efficiency.

Summary points

- Systematic reviews of treatments should include information on benefits and harms.
- Economic analyses should be developed using evidence on well-designed studies.
- The value of the benefits is difficult to establish without contingent valuations such as those from willingness to pay analyses.

References

1 Edmunds DK. *Dewhurst's Textbook of Obstetrics and Gynaecology for Post-Graduates, Sixth edition*. London: Blackwell Scientific, 1999.
2 Vessey MP, Villard-Mackintosh L, McPherson K, Coulter A, Yeates D. The epidemiology of hysterectomy: findings in a large cohort study. *Br J Obstet Gynaecol* 1992;**99**:402–7.
3 Stewart EA. Uterine fibroids. *Lancet* 2001;**357**:293–8.

4 Myers ER, Steege JF. Risk adjustment for complications of hysterectomy: limitations of routinely collected administrative data. *Am J Obstet Gynecol* 1999;**181**:567–75.
5 Lethaby A, Vollenhoven B, Sowter M. Preoperative GnRHa analogue therapy before hysterectomy or myomectomy for uterine fibroids. (Cochrane Review).*The Cochrane Library*, Issue 4. Oxford: Update Software, 2001.
6 Matta WH, Shaw RW, Nye M. Long-term follow-up of patients with uterine fibroids after treatment with the LHRH agonist buserelin. *Br J Obstet Gynaecol* 1989;**96**:200–6.
7 Stovall TG. Rationale for the short-term use of luteinising hormone-releasing hormone analogues in the treatment of uterine myomata. *Horm Res* 1989;**32** (Suppl 1):134–6.
8 Statistics New Zealand. *New Zealand Income Survey*. Wellington: Government of New Zealand, 2000.
9 Acien P, Quereda F. Abdominal myomectomy: results of a simple operative technique. *Fertil Steril* 1996;**65**:41–51.
10 Drummond M, Jefferson T. Guidelines for authors and peer reviewers of economic submissions to the BMJ. The BMJ Economic Evaluation Working Party. *BMJ* 1996;**313**:275–83.
11 Ryan M. Using willingness to pay to assess the benefits of assisted reproductive techniques. *Health Econ* 1996;**5**:543–58.
12 Torgerson DJ, Donaldson C, Russell IT, Reid DM. Hormone replacement therapy: compliance and cost after screening for osteoporosis. *Eur J Obstet Gynecol Reprod Biol* 1995;**59**:57–60.
13 Crowley P. Prophylactic corticosteroids for preterm birth. (Cochrane Review). *The Cochrane Library*, Issue 3. Oxford: Update Software, 2001.
14 The Albumin Reviewers. Human albumin solution for resuscitation and volume expansion in critically ill patients. (Cochrane Review). *The Cochrane Library*, Issue 4. Oxford: Update Software, 2001.
15 Maynard A, Kanavos P. Health economics: an evolving paradigm. *Health Econ* 2000;**9**:183–90.
16 NHS Executive. *Faster access to modern treatments: how NICE appraisal will work*. Leeds: Department of Health, 1999.

5: Evidence-based economic evaluation: how the use of different data sources can impact results

DOUGLAS COYLE, KAREN M LEE

Introduction

The practice of conducting economic evaluations through decision analysis based on secondary data sources has become well established.[1,2] However, it has been argued that economic analysis conducted through decision analysis is open to bias.[3] This is evident from certain journals questioning the scientific rigour of decision analysis-based studies.[4] Concerns over bias have been particularly pertinent to analysis funded by industry.[5]

The Economics Methods Group of the Cochrane Collaboration is one of many bodies interested in improving the "evidence base" of inputs used in economic analysis. By this, the choice of input parameters into decision analytic models would be based on standards pertaining to the quality and accuracy of data sources. The adoption of such standards may limit the potential for bias.

In a review of economic evaluations conducted in the field of osteoporosis, all analyses were conducted using forms of decision analytic modelling based on existing data. However, studies differed in their source of data inputs.[6] For example, a number of the studies identified obtained their estimates of effectiveness from single clinical trials rather than systematic reviews of all available trials.

The objective of this chapter is to demonstrate the effect of using alternative data sources for four key inputs into decision analysis-based economic analysis: clinical effect sizes, baseline risks, costs/resource use and utilities. Other inputs could have been considered (for example, compliance and duration of therapy). However, for brevity, the focus is on four of the most important data inputs which are common to all analysis.

Table 5.1 Levels of clinical evidence.

1++	High-quality meta-analyses, systematic reviews of RCTs, or RCTs with a very low risk of bias
1+	Well-conducted meta-analyses, systematic reviews of RCTs, or RCTs with a low risk of bias
1–	Meta-analyses, systematic reviews of RCTs, or RCTs with a high risk of bias
2++	High-quality systematic reviews of case control or cohort studies High-quality case control or cohort studies with a very low risk of confounding, bias, or chance and a high probability that the relationship is causal
2+	Well-conducted case control or cohort studies with a low risk of confounding, bias, or chance and a moderate probability that the relationship is causal
2–	Case control or cohort studies with a high risk of confounding, bias, or chance and a significant risk that the relationship is not causal
3	Non-analytic studies: for example, case reports, case series
4	Expert opinion

Source: Based on Sackett and others (Canadian Task Force on the Periodic Health Examination)[7]

The impact of different sources is assessed through analysis of the cost-effectiveness of alendronate compared to no therapy in the treatment of postmenopausal women with osteoporosis.

Different sources of data

Previous guidance

There is broad agreement with the levels of evidence of clinical effectiveness, as suggested by Sackett and others, which have become a tenet of evidence-based medicine (Table 5.1).[7] Within this hierarchy of evidence, there is a clear statement in favour of the use of randomised controlled trials over observational data sources such as case control or cohort studies.

There is a lack of a similar hierarchy regarding the levels of evidence about resource use, costs and value of outcomes which should be used to populate decision analyses for the conduct of economic analyses. Sackett and others have also proposed levels of economic evidence (Table 5.2).[8] However, there are a number of potential problems with this hierarchy. There is no consideration of either the timing of the analysis, and the generalisability of studies across geographical and political areas is ignored. The hierarchy also mixes such disparate issues as assessment of methodological quality and decision rules in acceptance or rejection of the treatment evaluated. More importantly, the proposed hierarchy focuses primarily on standards for economic analysis for use in decision making and not standards for the source of data inputs for economic analysis.

What is necessary is an attempt to identify specific factors relating to data sources for key parameters that determine their appropriateness for the analysis at hand. In the following sections, four key data parameters are discussed and the specific features of potential data sources that need to be considered are highlighted.

Table 5.2 Levels of economic evidence.

1++	Systematic review of level 1 economic studies
1+	Analysis comparing all (critically validated) alternative outcomes against appropriate cost measurement, and including a sensitivity analysis incorporating clinically sensible variations in important variables
1−	Clearly as good or better, but cheaper. Clearly as bad or worse but more expensive. Clearly better or worse at the same cost
2++	SR (with homogeneity) of Level ≥ 2 economic studies
2+	Analysis comparing a limited number of alternative outcomes against appropriate cost measurement, and including a sensitivity analysis incorporating clinically sensible variations in important variables. Analysis without accurate cost measurement, but including a sensitivity analysis incorporating clinically sensible variations in important variables.
3	Analysis with no sensitivity analysis
4	Expert opinion without explicit critical appraisal, or based on economic theory

Source: From Phillips *et al*[8] (Centre for Evidence-based Medicine), http://cebm.jr2.ox.ac.uk/docs/levels.html

Clinical effect sizes

For economic analysis, the source of clinical effect sizes of comparator drugs may be the most crucial data input. The hierarchy for clinical evidence proposed by Sackett does in some way help in assessing the relative quality of potential data sources for effect sizes; demonstrating clear support for meta-analyses over individual clinical trials over observational studies. However, there are many aspects of randomised controlled trials which may make it difficult to incorporate such data in economic analyses.

The preponderance of placebo controlled trials is a major problem and is associated with a lack of head to head studies between the relevant comparator therapies within an analysis. Thus, many studies require the computation of synthetic comparisons between comparators through comparison of the results of placebo controlled trials. This requires that trial designs be similar, especially in relation to patient characteristics and inclusion/exclusion criteria for the data to be appropriate for economic evaluations.

A further problem relates to the use of intermediate endpoints rather than final outcomes. For example, in trials of osteoporosis therapies the principal outcome of interest is, generally, either changes in the patient's bone mineral density or changes in fracture rates. For both outcomes, within an economic analysis the requirements will be to forecast long-term survival, quality of life and costs based on the clinical effect sizes. Fracture-based models have been designed and validated in terms of the forecasting of long-term outcomes. However, analysis based on bone mineral density will have to first incorporate a model predicting fracture rates based on changes in bone mineral density before forecasting such long-term outcomes. The validity of bone mineral density as a predictor of fracture rates whilst on bisphosphonates has been questioned.

The problems outlined above are pertinent to clinical reviews that do not incorporate economic analysis. However, the focus of this chapter is only on their impact on economic analysis. Given the above, it is clear that not all randomised trials can be considered appropriate sources for effect sizes for economic analysis.

Baseline risks of clinical events

The guidelines by Sackett have much less relevance with respect to the source for data on the baseline risks of clinical events. Characteristics of clinical trials, especially patient inclusion/exclusion criteria, can lead to the incidence of clinical events such as fracture being much different than would be experienced in normal clinical practice. Clinical trial populations are often a select group of patients for which the incidence of events may be substantially lower or higher than the norm. In addition, the design of trial protocols often influences the detection of clinical events, leading to an overestimate of their baseline incidence.

Given concerns with trial-based data, a preferred source for baseline risk data is likely to be the analysis of good quality administrative or epidemiological databases. However, the question of what entails good quality administrative data is less clear, but involves consideration of the level of bias and accuracy and generalisability to broader populations.

Event rates can vary by geographical and political areas because of a number of factors, primarily because of the prevailing prevalence of risk factors (for example, genetic predisposition, diet, exercise, climate). Given this, bias may be introduced into analyses based on databases from different locations. For example, fracture rates are greater in Canada than elsewhere. Hence, a UK analysis incorporating Canadian baseline rates would bias results in favour of active therapy.

Costs and resource use

In the measurement of resource use, the major potential data sources include prospective data collection within randomised controlled trials and observational studies, the retrospective analysis of randomised controlled trials and observational studies and analysis of administrative databases. In the measurement of unit costs, potential sources include prospective costing or analysis of administrative databases. In addition, for both costs and resource use, some studies have merely used data from previous studies or from Delphi panel estimates.

Delphi panels and previous studies may be seen as the least preferred sources, primarily through concerns of accuracy and relevance. However, the other, previously mentioned, sources of data all have potential problems that need to be considered within each individual study.

In measuring resource use through either trials or other sources, it is necessary to consider the generalisability of the data source to the broader patient population. For clinical trial data, this relates to the degree that both the patient population and clinical practice within the trial relate to practice within the whole population considered in the economic analysis. For administrative data sources, this relates to the inclusive nature of the database (both geographical and clinical) and whether it can accurately identify all relevant patients and related resource use.

In addition to the above, it should be emphasized that because of the substantive differences between jurisdictions in terms of clinical practice and health care financing, it is preferable if not essential that data sources from the geographic or political area to which the study relates be employed in analysis. Otherwise, detailed sensitivity analyses around such estimates are required.

Utilities

There is a lack of consensus over the preferred source of utility values to be used in economic analysis. Such lack of consensus relates to the preferred tools for utility elicitation and the preferred source for the estimation of utility values.[9,10]

Despite this lack of consensus it may be possible to distinguish in terms of appropriateness between the use of utilities from studies specifically designed for the particular analysis and utility estimates derived from previously published sources or from Delphi panel estimates. In addition, given that there is some evidence that there may be cultural differences in utility values placed on health states, preference should be given to sources of utilities relating to the geographic or political area to which the study relates.[11]

Potential hierarchies

Given the above, Table 5.3 details potential hierarchies for data sources. The hierarchies provide a list of potential data sources for each data component discussed above, with a potential ranking of their appropriateness. Sources are ranked on an increasing scale, with the most appropriate sources given a rank of 1. The ranking highlights how different data sources are appropriate for different data components. It is emphasized that these should not be considered as a consensus statement but rather a template from which appropriate hierarchies could be developed.

Analysis of impact of different sources

In this section, the analysis conducted to assess the impact on the results of an economic analysis of alternative sources for the key four variables listed above is outlined.

Model

The model adopted for this analysis is similar to a previous analysis of the cost-effectiveness of alternative drug therapies for the treatment of postmenopausal women.[12] Economic analysis was conducted within a

Table 5.3 Potential hierarchies of data sources for economic analyses.

A	*Clinical effect sizes*
1++	Meta-analysis of RCTs with direct comparison between comparator therapies, measuring final outcomes
1+	Single RCT with direct comparison between comparator therapies, measuring final outcomes
2++	Meta-analysis of RCTs with direct comparison between comparator therapies, measuring surrogate outcomes Meta-analysis of placebo controlled RCTs with similar trial populations, measuring final outcomes for each individual therapy
2+	Single RCT with direct comparison between comparator therapies, measuring surrogate outcomes Single placebo controlled RCTs with similar trial populations, measuring final outcomes for each individual therapy
3++	Meta-analysis of placebo controlled RCTs with similar trial populations, surrogate outcomes for each individual therapy
3+	Single placebo controlled RCTs with similar trial populations, measuring final outcomes for each individual therapy
4	Case control or cohort studies
5	Non-analytic studies, for example, case reports, case series
6	Expert opinion
B	*Baseline clinical data*
1++	Case series or analysis of reliable administrative databases specifically conducted for the study covering patients solely from the jurisdiction of interest
1+	Recent case series or analysis of reliable administrative databases covering patients solely from the jurisdiction of interest
2	Recent case series or analysis of reliable administrative databases covering patients from another jurisdiction
3	Old case series or analysis of reliable administrative databases Estimates from RCTs
4	Estimates from previously published economic analyses: unsourced
5	Expert opinion
C	*Resource use*
1++	Prospective data collection or analysis of reliable administrative data for specific study
1+	Recently published results of prospective data collection or recent analysis of reliable administrative data – same jurisdiction
2++	Unsourced data from previous economic evaluations – same jurisdiction
2+	Recently published results of prospective data collection or recent analysis of reliable administrative data – different jurisdiction
3	Unsourced data from previous economic evaluations – different jurisdiction
4	Expert opinion
D	*Costs*
1++	Cost calculations based on reliable databases or data sources conducted for specific study – same jurisdiction
1+	Recently published cost calculations based on reliable databases or data sources – same jurisdiction
2++	Unsourced data from previous economic evaluations – same jurisdiction
2+	Recently published cost calculations based on reliable databases or data sources – different jurisdiction

Continued

Table 5.3 (Continued)

3	Unsourced data from previous economic evaluations – different jurisdiction
4	Expert opinion
E	*Utilities*
1	Direct utility assessment for the specific study from a sample either: (a) of the general population (b) with knowledge of the disease(s) of interest (c) of patients with the disease(s) of interest Indirect utility assessment for specific study from patient sample with disease(s) of interest; using a tool validated for the patient population
2	Direct utility assessment from a previous study from a sample either: (a) of the general population (b) with knowledge of the disease(s) of interest (c) of patients with the disease(s) of interest Indirect utility assessment from a previous study from patient sample with disease(s) of interest; using a tool validated for the patient population
3	Indirect utility assessment from a patient sample with disease(s) of interest; using a tool not validated for the patient population Patient preference values obtained from a visual analogue scale
4	Delphi panels, expert opinion

Markov model based within an Excel spreadsheet with results pertinent to 65-year-old women on therapy for five years with allowance for an estimate of patients' compliance with therapy.

The clinical effectiveness of each therapy was assessed by estimating the associated relative risk reductions for hip, wrist and vertebral fractures based on a meta-analysis of all published randomised controlled trials. The baseline population risk of fracture was estimated through analysis of administrative databases.

This study focuses on the analysis of alendronate compared to no therapy, for which there is the most clinical trial data. In the published paper, based on a meta-analysis of all available clinical trials, alendronate led to an incremental cost per quality-adjusted life year (QALY) gained, compared to no therapy, of Can$47 800.[12]

Source of clinical effect size

Conducting analysis based on the results of a single clinical trial may allow analysts to bias the results in favour or against a particular intervention. Analysis based on the results of meta-analysis can be argued to provide both a more exact estimate of the treatment effect and a more precise estimate in terms of narrower confidence intervals, whilst at the same time reducing the potential for accusations of bias.[13]

To assess the potential impact of using individual trials rather than a meta-analysis, the analysis above was repeated using effect sizes from three of the trials as these provided relative risks for hip, wrist and vertebral fractures for alendronate.[14–16] Analysis was conducted using Crystal Ball simulation software which allows the conduct of Monte

Carlo probabilistic analysis. For each variable in the decision model a probability distribution was derived either through use of confidence intervals and other data from clinical trials and the utility assessments or through assumptions relating to the size of standard deviations associated with cost estimates. For the simulation analysis, 10 000 simulations were conducted, whereby 10 000 outcome estimates were obtained by rerunning the model employing a different value for each data input randomly selected from that variable's probability distribution.

A 95% credible interval around the incremental cost per QALY can be constructed which represents the 2·5 and 97·5 percentile of the distribution of the outcome measure.[17] Given the convincing arguments relating to the irrelevance of standard statistical testing for cost-effectiveness ratios, the proportions of simulations with a cost per QALY greater than Can$ 100 000 are presented. This can be seen as a rudimentary measure of the concern of decision makers for more sample information to inform the choice they have to make: that is, whether a decision should be made or whether it should be deferred until more information is available.[18]

Source of baseline clinical event data

In the published study, the risks of fractures were determined through analysis of administrative databases recording physician visits and hospitalisations by diagnosis within Canada. To assess the impact of different sources of baseline risks of clinical events, analysis was repeated using event rates from non-Canadian cohort studies and from a UK economic study which used event rates from a single clinical trial.[15,19–22]

Source of utilities

In the published study, utility values for relevant health states were derived from an ongoing study in Ottawa[23] related to fracture using direct utility assessment methods. To assess the impact of different sources of utility values on the results of analysis, analysis was repeated using utility values derived from a US study using direct methods and from a UK economic study which used hypothetical valuations based on indirect utility assessment.[22,24]

Source of cost data

In the published study, costs associated with fractures were derived from two recent Canadian studies which estimated costs based on the analysis of routine administrative databases. Analysis was repeated using alternative estimates of costs from Canada and from previous studies from different jurisdictions, inflated and converted to Canadian dollars.[22,25–29]

Results

Source of clinical effect size

Table 5.4 provides estimates of the cost per QALY gained for alendronate based on the three individual trials and the meta-analysis.

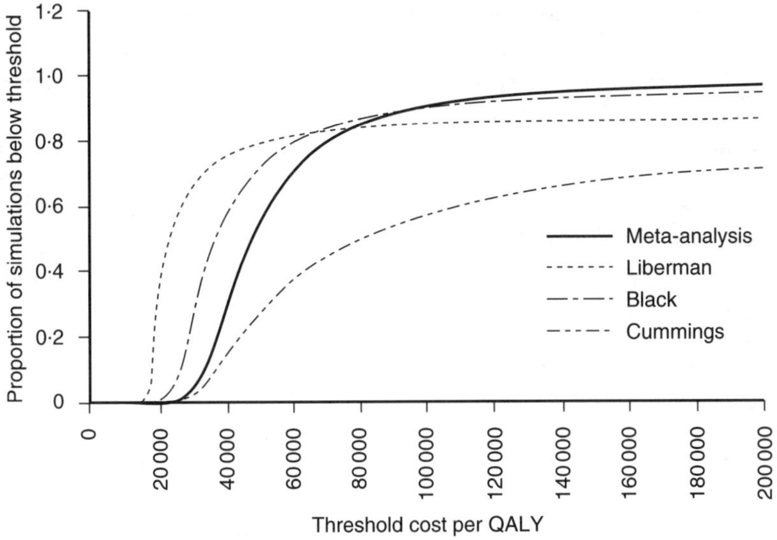

Threshold cost per QALY relates to the maximum willingness of a decision maker to pay for an additional QALY gain
The proportion of simulations below the threshold is the proportion of the replications from the Monte Carlo analysis which are below the threshold cost per QALY

Figure 5.1 Cumulative distributions of cost per QALY for alendronate.

Estimates of the cost per QALY based on the individual trials ranged from Can$23 700 to Can$78 700 compared to the estimate from the meta-analysis of Can$47 800.

For the Monte Carlo simulation exercise 10 000 simulations were conducted based on the confidence intervals for each of the three clinical trials and for the meta-analysis of all relevant trials. Observations for the incremental cost per QALY are illustrated in Figure 5.1. It is evident that the curves in the figure cross, which demonstrates the effect of the magnitude of the confidence intervals around the clinical effect sizes. The proportions of simulations with a cost per QALY greater than Can$100 000 are detailed in Table 5.4.

Source of baseline clinical event data

Analysis based on event rates from the clinical trial led to a cost per QALY gained figure of Can$27 800. Analysis based on non-Canadian population databases estimated a cost per QALY of Can$154 600.

Utilities

The estimated cost per QALY based on analysis using utility values from the US study was Can$46 300. Analysis based on hypothetical values from the UK study found a cost per QALY of Can$54 700.

Table 5.4 Cost per QALY based on different data sources (Canadian $).

	Cost per QALY	
Base case	47 800	(10·0%)
Clinical effect size (individual trials)		
Liberman[14]	23 700	(15·5%)
Black[15]	37 200	(10·2%)
Cummings[16]	78 700	(43·2%)
Alternative source of baseline clinical data		
Clinical trial[15,24]	27 800	
Non-Canadian data[19–21]	154 600	
Alternative utility values		
US direct methods[23]	46 300	
UK hypothetical values[24]	54 700	
Alternate sources of cost data		
Other Canadian[25]	45 800	
UK[24]	51 800	
Norway[26]	44 600	
Australia[27]	51 500	
Denmark[28]	50 000	
United States[29]	48 300	

Figures in parentheses are percentage of simulations for which cost per QALY is greater than $100 000

Source of cost data

Analysis based on the alternative Canadian estimates of costs produced a cost per QALY of $45 800. Analyses based on the non-Canadian sources obtained a range of cost per QALY estimates from $44 600 to $51 800.

Discussion

The potential to bias resulting through the use of different sources of data is apparent with the results of the analysis. However, the results appeared to confirm that it is uncertainty over the appropriate source of clinical data, be it effect sizes or baseline risks, which has most impact on the results of the analysis.

The estimated cost per QALY gained based on effect sizes from the individual trials varied considerably. Results based on the meta-analysis appeared to represent a more central estimate implying a less biased result. Thus, it should not be assumed that all analyses conducted based on single trials are necessarily biased: rather, that there is the potential for bias (either implicit or explicit). However, deliberate bias can be introduced to both favour the particular therapy or to make the therapy appear less attractive compared to an alternative therapy.

Results also varied considerably by whether the baseline risk of fracture was based on clinical trial event rates or event rates from administrative data sets. Given the atypical nature of trial settings, the baseline risk of events from trials may be inappropriate for economic analysis. Thus, analysis based on data from non-selective populations may be more appropriate provided that the data are accurate and reflective of the population as a whole. However, results of this analysis suggest that in certain instances such data may have to be country-specific given the sizable differences in results based on Canadian and non-Canadian data.

As economists become more concerned with the applicability of their analyses, any initiatives to reduce accusations of bias should be welcomed. Thus, it can be argued that in future economic analyses based on re-analysis of secondary data, estimates of clinical effectiveness should be based on meta-analysis of all existing trials and estimates of the baseline risk of events should be based on accurate "real world" data. Concern over the sources of costs and utility data, while important, should be considered less serious than concern over clinical inputs.

Summary points

- In the interpretation of clinical data, there are generally agreed standards relating to the quality of research evidence. However, there is a lack of agreement over what constitutes good evidence for specific data points in economic evaluation. This chapter considered alternative levels of data quality relating to clinical effects, resource use and quality of life/utilities and their impact on results was illustrated by an evaluation of treatments for osteoporosis.
- When modelling cost-effectiveness by use of different estimates of clinical effects, baseline risks, costs and utility estimates, the case study used in this chapter shows that cost per QALY varies most according to which estimate of clinical outcome is used.
- Economic analysis conducted through decision analytic techniques has been open to criticism over the ease with which desired results can be obtained. In this study, it has been demonstrated that results can vary widely based on the data source employed. The adoption of standards for assessing the quality of data inputs based on an evidence-based approach may reduce the level of criticism.

References

1 Buxton MJ, Drummond MF, Van Hout BA, Prince RL, Sheldon TA, Szucs T *et al.* Modelling in economic evaluation: an unavoidable fact of life. *Health Econ* 1997;**6**:217–27.
2 Jefferson T, Mugford M, Gray A, Demicheli V. An exercise on the feasibility of carrying out secondary economic analyses. *Health Econ* 1996;**5**:155–65.
3 Freemantle N, Maynard A. Something rotten in the state of clinical and economic evaluations? *Health Econ* 1994;**3**:63–7.
4 Kassirer JP, Angell M. The journal's policy on cost-effectiveness analyses. *N Engl J Med* 1994;**331**:669–70.
5 Hillman AL, Eisenberg JM, Pauly MV, Bloom BS, Glick H, Kinosian B *et al.* Avoiding bias in the conduct and reporting of cost-effectiveness research sponsored by pharmaceutical companies. *N Engl J Med* 1991;**324**:1362–5.

6 Cranney A, Coyle D, Welch V, Lee KM, Tugwell P. A review of economic evaluation in osteoporosis. *Arthritis Care Res* 1999;**12**:425–34.
7 Canadian Task Force on the Periodic Health Examination. The periodic health examination. *Can Med Assoc J* 1979;**121**:1193–254.
8 Phillips B *et al.* Levels of evidence and grades of recommendations. NHS research and development centre for evidence-based medicine, 5 pages. (http://cebm.jr2.ox.ac.uk/docs/levels.html).
9 Drummond MF, O'Brien B, Stoddart GL, Torrance GW. *Methods for the economic evaluation of health care programmes.* Oxford: Oxford University Press, 1997.
10 Gold M, Siegel JE, Russell LB, Weinstein MC. *Cost-effectiveness in health and medicine.* Oxford: Oxford University Press, 1996.
11 Coyle D, Maunsell E, Wells G, Graham I, Lee KM, Meunier N, Peterson JE. Differences in preference values between cultural groups: women's preferences over lifetime risks associated with postmenopausal osteoporosis therapy. Annual Meeting of the International Society of Technology Assessment in Health Care, 1999;**15**:81.
12 Coyle D, Cranney A, Lee KM, Welch V, Tugwell P. Cost effectiveness of nasal calcitonin in postmenopausal women: use of Cochrane Collaboration methods for meta-analysis within economic evaluation. *Pharmacoeconomics* 2001;**19**:565–75.
13 Sacks HS, Berrier J, Reitman D, Ancona-Berk VA, Chalmers TC. Meta-analyses of randomized controlled trials. *N Engl J Med* 1987;**316**:450–5.
14 Liberman UA, Weiss SR, Broll J, Minne HW, Quan H, Bell NH *et al.* Effect of oral alendronate on bone mineral density and the incidence of fractures in postmenopausal osteoporosis. The Alendronate Phase III Osteoporosis Treatment Study Group. *N Engl J Med* 1995;**333**:1437–43.
15 Black DM, Cummings SR, Karpf DB, Cauley JA, Thompson DE, Nevitt MC *et al.* Randomised trial of effect of alendronate on risk of fracture in women with existing vertebral fractures. Fracture Intervention Trial Research Group. *Lancet* 1996;**348**: 1535–41.
16 Cummings SR, Black DM, Thompson DE, Applegate WB, Barrett-Connor E, Musliner TA *et al.* Effect of alendronate on risk of fracture in women with low bone density but without vertebral fractures: results from the Fracture Intervention Trial. *JAMA* 1998;**280**:2077–82.
17 Spiegelhalter DJ, Myles JP, Jones DR, Abrams KR. Bayesian methods in health technology assessment: a review. *Health Technol Assess* 2000;**4**:1–130.
18 Claxton K. The irrelevance of inference: a decision-making approach to the stochastic evaluation of health care technologies. *J Health Econ* 1999;**18**:341–64.
19 Kannus P, Parkkari J, Sievanen H, Heinonen A, Vuori I, Jarvinen M. Epidemiology of hip fractures. *Bone* 1996;**18**:57S–63S.
20 Karagas MR, Lu-Yao GL, Barrett JA, Beach ML, Baron JA. Heterogeneity of hip fracture: age, race, sex, and geographic patterns of femoral neck and trochanteric fractures among the US elderly. *Am J Epidemiol* 1996;**143**:677–82.
21 Donaldson LJ, Cook A, Thomson RG. Incidence of fractures in a geographically defined population. *J Epidemiol Comm Health* 1990;**44**:241–5.
22 Best L, Milne R. Bisphosphonates (alendronate and etidronate) in the management of osteoporosis. DEC Report No. 79. Wessex Institute for Health Research and Development, 1998.
23 Cranney A, Coyle D, Pham BA, Tetroe J, Wells G, Jolly E *et al.* The psychometric properties of patient preferences in osteoporosis. *J Rheumatol* 2001;**28**:132–7.
24 Silverman S, Simons R. Utility values for osteoporosis outcomes. Personal communication, 2001.
25 Goeree R, O'Brien B, Pettitt D, Cuddy L, Ferraz M, Adachi J. An assessment of the burden of illness due to osteoporosis in Canada. *SOGC* 1996;**Suppl**:15–22.
26 Kristiansen IS, Falch JA, Andersen L, Aursnes I. [Use of alendronate in osteoporosis–is it cost-effective?]. *Tidsskr Nor Laegeforen* 1997;**117**:2619–22.
27 Cheung AP, Wren BG. A cost-effectiveness analysis of hormone replacement therapy in the menopause. *Med J Aust* 1992;**156**:312–16.
28 Ankjaer-Jensen A, Johnell O. Prevention of osteoporosis: cost-effectiveness of different pharmaceutical treatments. *Osteoporosis Int* 1996;**6**:265–75.
29 Tosteson AN, Weinstein MC. Cost-effectiveness of hormone replacement therapy after the menopause. *Baillieres Clin Obstet Gynaecol* 1991;**5**:943–59.

6: Methodological quality of economic evaluations of health care interventions – evidence from systematic reviews

TOM JEFFERSON, LUKE VALE, VITTORIO DEMICHELI

Introduction

Evidence-based decision making has never been so complex, despite increased availability of large amounts of information on all aspects of health care. One of the most important aspects of decision making in a resource-limited world is the opportunity costs of investing resources in particular interventions or programmes. To enable rational and ethical decisions to be made in health care, good information on at least two closely linked aspects of interventions (effectiveness and efficiency) are required. Studies assessing effectiveness (the analysis of the effects of interventions in terms of changes in clinical indices, health status or some wider notion of benefits) have increased considerably in the past decade. Such studies are either "primary", often randomised controlled trials (RCTs), or of synthesis design (usually systematic reviews of RCTs). In the past two decades there has also been similar considerable growth in economic evaluations, studies assessing the efficiency of interventions.[1,2] However, greater quantity may not necessarily mean better quality, especially given that assessment of efficiency is heavily dependent on a range of estimates, incorporated in the evaluation, such as those of the effects of the intervention being evaluated (see for example Chapter 5 by Coyle and Lee).

A number of reviews carried out and published in the period 1990–94 illustrated to the research community and decision makers the variability of quality of methods employed by authors of economic evaluations and their poor reporting.[3] Similarly, a survey of editorial practices in general and specialist medical journals described the absence of editorial policies in place to assess economic evaluations prior to publication.[4,5]

These findings led to a series of initiatives aimed at increasing the homogeneity and quality of economic evaluations and their reporting. The first of these initiatives was the production of guidelines for carrying out and submitting economic evaluations to regulatory and reimbursement bodies. Such guidelines were introduced in Australia before being taken up by other agencies such as, and most notably, the Canadian Coordinating Office of Health Technology Assessment and the UK's National Institute for Clinical Excellence. A second initiative was the establishment of a working party with the express aim of developing guidelines for submission and editorial management of economic evaluation in medical journals of the *BMJ* group. While such guidelines were intended to improve the quality of primary research they have been used, as is illustrated below, to consider the quality of published primary studies. Finally, there has been further research into the general topic of the quality of economic evaluation methods. A glance through any of the main journals for health economics, health services research or health technology assessment shows that such research has covered the whole spectrum of methodological issues relating to the conduct of economic evaluation. The systematic reviews that form the basis of this review are also indicative of the breadth and depth of this research.

In this chapter the aim is to assess the evidence on the quality of methods and reporting of economic evaluations of health care interventions. The assessment is based on the findings of systematic reviews of economic evaluations carried out in the period 1990–2000. Comments are also made on the evidence of the effect of interventions such as guidelines, editorial policies and checklists for the conduct of economic evaluations carried out in the last decade of the old millennium to assess the effectiveness and efficiency of health care interventions and so inform decisions about licensing and provision. If these initiatives were successful one would expect signs of an impact on overall methodological quality.

Methods

A search for systematic reviews was carried out. Systematic reviews were defined as attempts to rigorously identify and synthesise all economic evaluations in the stated jurisdiction (such as methodological aspects or clinical areas) of the review. To be included, potential systematic reviews had to report a structured search strategy for the systematic identification of original studies. This included details of the databases searched, the years searched and details of the keywords and MeSH terms used. Also required was a description of how the studies (which for some studies did not just mean economic evaluation) were chosen to be included in the systematic review. Finally, reviews were only included if they provided detailed descriptions about how the quality of economic evaluations was assessed.

The search for systematic reviews covered several private and public electronic databases and a hand search of issues of *Health Economics* from 1992 to the end of 2000. Full details of the search, methods and findings can be found in the text of our paper "The quality of systematic reviews of economic evaluations in healthcare".[6]

One or more reviewers examined each retrieved citation for relevance and those thought to be so were obtained in full. Two reviewers then compared each study against the selection criteria independently, resolving disagreements by discussion. For each included systematic review the following descriptive data was first extracted as follows: author(s) and year of study; topic and study question; design (for example, cost-benefit analysis) and number of included economic evaluations; year of publication or preparation of included economic evaluations; instrument used to assess quality of included economic evaluations; and main study conclusions (see Appendix 6.1).

Studies that met inclusion criteria were quality-scored for methods employed using the following criteria adapted from Oxman *et al*,[7,8] and Mulrow and Cook.[9]

A Did the review address a focused question?
B Is it unlikely that important relevant studies were missed?
C Were the inclusion criteria used to select articles appropriate?
D Was the validity of the included studies assessed?
E Was the assessment of studies reproducible?
F Were the design and/or methods and/or topic of included studies broadly comparable?
G How reproducible are the overall results?
H Will the results help resource allocation in health care?

Each stem was answered by one of the following items (with corresponding score): Impossible to judge (1); No (2); Partly (3); Yes (4). The scores for each of the eight stems (A to H) were then averaged to obtain an overall score for the reviewer. As this was a subjective exercise, a calculation was made of Spearman's rank-order correlation coefficient, correlating inter-reviewer agreement. Spearman's coefficient is a measure of association between two variables requiring that both variables be measured in at least an ordinal scale, so that objects or individuals under study may be ranked in two ordered series.

Systematic reviews were also grouped by the broad questions or issues they were addressing. Thus, reviews were classified according to whether they assessed either general methodological quality of economic evaluations in health care or specific interventions (for example, interventions to prevent HIV infection), or by the economic study design included (for example, cost-benefit analysis, or cost-utility analysis) or by specific methods used in economic evaluations included in the review (for example, contingent valuation, costing).

It should be noted that the work presented here is in progress. Further relevant reviews will be sought and assessed to summarise the methodological quality of the studies they contain.

Two reviewers extracted data on methods of assessing the quality of economic evaluations included in each of the methodological reviews in the study. In order to facilitate a comparison across the included systematic reviews, the method that each included review used to assess the quality of economic evaluations that they contained was compared to the 35 criteria provided by the *BMJ* checklist for editors and authors of economic evaluations. If the included review assessed the same methodological aspect (for example, was the viewpoint of the analysis stated?) as a *BMJ* checklist criterion a "Yes" response was assigned and if it did not cover that criterion then a "No" response was assigned. One exception to this is when it was unclear whether a particular *BMJ* criterion was covered, in which case a "Not Clear" (NC) response was assigned. The final exception was made for reviews that focused on a specific methodological aspect such as a particular method of benefit assessment. In these cases a "Not Applicable" (NA) response was assigned for those criteria not relevant to the question addressed by the included review (see Appendix 6.2).

Two reviewers extracted findings on the quality of the economic evaluations included in each methodological study. These are summarised under the following headings: study design; assessment of benefits; assessment of costs; analysis; and conclusions (see Appendix 6.3, Appendix 6.4).

Results

A total of 37 study reports that could satisfy inclusion criteria were identified. Of these, 18 failed to meet the inclusion criteria and were excluded from further analysis. The remaining 19 reports are summarised below.

Findings – the quality of systematic reviews

A summary of the findings is presented in Appendix 6.1. Despite the subjective nature of the quality assessment used, there was inter-rater agreement (with Spearman's RHO ranging from 1 to 0·989 for the eight quality items). The vast majority of included reviews scored very highly in the quality assessment of their methods, making their conclusions more credible. It is also more likely that good reporting practices can be equated with good methods of conducting the reviews. A common problem was the use of different instruments for quality assessment of the economic evaluations that were incorporated in each of the systematic reviews. Although this finding may raise concerns about the comparability of the results of the included reviews, it is not surprising, as there is no recognised evaluation instrument and each review assessed slightly different methodological aspects of economic evaluations. To enhance comparability of the results of the reviews the quality criteria used in each review were mapped and compared with those in the *BMJ* checklist (see below).

Findings – the quality of economic evaluations assessed in the systematic reviews

Although the reviews can furnish only a partial picture with possible duplicate inclusion of some economic evaluations, the consistent findings are of variable quality of methodology and of possible slow improvement. The impact of the initiatives taken to raise the quality of economic literature appears to have been, at best, slight. A recurring number of methodological flaws are evident in the economic evaluations assessed by the included reviews. To further explore the nature of the methodological weaknesses of the economic evaluations (summarised in the seventh column of Appendix 6.1) a more detailed review was also performed of the 19 included reviews. The findings of each review were grouped using the *BMJ* checklist.[3] The summary of the quality of studies assessed in the reviews was divided into five broad categories corresponding to specific items on the *BMJ* checklist (see Appendix 6.2):

- The approach – items 1 to 7
- The assessment of effectiveness/benefits – items 8 to 13
- The assessment of resource use/costs – items 14 to 19
- Methods of analysis – items 20 to 32
- Conclusions – items 22 to 35

The extent to which the quality criteria used by the reviews to assess the included economic evaluations could be mapped against the *BMJ* guidelines is shown in Appendix 6.2. As can be seen, the quality criteria covered by each individual review varied. To some extent this was because, as already stated, each review had a specific objective, making it at times inappropriate to assess all aspects of quality. Some reviews were focused on specific aspects of economic evaluation methodology and carried out assessments far more specific and detailed than those covered in the *BMJ* guidelines (for example Brazier *et al*[10]).

Although the extent and nature of coverage of quality assessment varied considerably, a number of key points based on the summaries of the findings of each individual study presented in Appendix 6.3 and Appendix 6.4 stand out. First, in almost all aspects covered by quality assessment the economic evaluations included in the systematic reviews identified were, in general, found wanting. Second, a number of the included reviews commented on lack of clarity of study questions and consequent viewpoint of the analysis and variability of epidemiological assumptions used in the evaluation.

These are arguably major flaws, which are not specific to economic study designs. Third, the conceptual and decision making context of the evaluation is, at best, unclear. This confusion is probably reflected in the variability of application of economic study designs (and classification confusion), also commented upon by the reviewers. Fourth, studies tended to lack clear descriptions of methods of estimation of effectiveness of interventions, utilities, benefits, resource use and costs. Basic calculation errors in a significant minority of studies were also discovered when the actual spreadsheets used in individual evaluations were checked.[11] Fifth, the reviews found that there was variability in the assumptions underlying the choice and origin of estimates of effect of the interventions evaluated. Last, the provision of descriptive information like the perspective of the analysis and price base, while lacking in many evaluations, may be improving over time; see for example the two Gerard studies[12,13] and that by Neumann.[14] However, potentially more useful information relating to the justification of specific practices, like the choice of discount rate, or the perspective taken were often not provided.[13] Similarly, key parts of economic methodology such as sensitivity analysis were more likely to be performed in more recent evaluations. However, much of this analysis may not be appropriate to the type of uncertainty faced.[15]

Several reviews remarked that the conclusions of a sizeable proportion of economic evaluations could not be justified on the basis of methods used. Thus, a section of economic literature representing over 1000 evaluations of different interventions and of different designs and carried out over different periods showed considerable methodological flaws, including variability of quality of incorporated estimates of effect. The results of this review appear to be insensitive to the quality of the methods used in the systematic reviews and the topic assessed.

Conclusions

The findings at this stage represent work in progress carried out within a Cochrane review of the quality of systematic reviews of economic evaluations. However, the evidence presented here points unequivocally to major gaps in the conduct and reporting of economic evaluations. A number of gaps can be identified. First, is the continued lack of clear descriptions of methodology. Second, is the lack of explanation and justification for the framework and approach used. Third, the quality of estimates of effectiveness of the interventions evaluated needs to be improved. While it is possible that single RCTs or reviews of RCTs may not have been available at the time of the conduct of the economic evaluation, a significant minority of evaluations rely on estimates of effect derived from single, small, non-randomised studies or, possibly even worse, expert opinion.

The current low level of quality of the literature, while not confined to this field alone, risks bringing health economics into disrepute among some decision makers and editors and feeds the scepticism of those who regard economics as a black art.

To address this problem the following initiatives are proposed:

- The definition, validation and acceptance of a standardised instrument for methodological quality assessment of economic evaluations and variants to assess specific economic methods (for example, contingent valuation or health status measurement).
- The monitoring of the methodological quality of economic evaluations using the standardised instrument, perhaps through a rolling survey with a two-year sampling frame starting from a set date, say 1990.
- The monitoring of unpublished populations of economic evaluations submitted to regulatory or reimbursement agencies (such as the UK's National Institute for Clinical Excellence) using the standardised instrument.
- Continued monitoring of the quality of systematic reviews of economic evaluations.
- The definition of a methodological research agenda to define best practice in systematic reviewing of economic evaluations.
- The preparation and maintenance of a specialised register of studies of methodological aspects of economic evaluations.
- The definition and acceptance by editors, regulators and research commissioners of clear policies to ensure quality of evaluations, preferably based on the standardised instrument.

Of course, economists are working towards some, even all, of the above. This is important if evidence-based health economics is to be taken seriously.

Summary points

Evidence from systematic reviews shows several major methodological flaws in published and unpublished economic evaluations:

- Lack of clear descriptions of methodology.
- Lack of explanation and justification for the framework and approach used.
- Low quality of estimates of effectiveness of the interventions evaluated.

Editors, research commissioners and regulators must take urgent steps to address the situation.

Appendices

Appendix 6.1 Summary of content of studies included in the review.

Study (first author and year)	Topic and study question	Mean quality score	Design (number) of included economic evaluations	Year of publication/ preparation of included economic evaluations	Instrument used to assess quality of primary studies	Main study conclusions
Adams 1992[16]	Assessment of quality of economic evaluations nested in RCTs	4·0	CBA and CEA (51)	1973–88	Ad hoc checklists: quality and completeness score (0 to 1)	There is considerable room for methodological improvement
Anonymous unpublished[17]	Assessment of quality of Spanish economic evaluations	3·25	CBA, CEA, CMA and CUA (87)	1983–99	Mixed 16-item classification/ quality checklist	Several methodological problems which appear to be similar to those in international reviews of the topic
Barber 1998[18]	Quality of statistic evaluation of cost data in RCTs	3·93	Not stated (45)	1995	Data extraction checklist based on statistical principles	Strong inferential conclusions made without supporting data
Brazier 1999[10]	Quality of HSM used in included studies	3·93	CCA and CUA (13)	1995	Checklist with three questions	Choice of instruments and their validity is unclear or questionable in 50% of studies
Demicheli 1997[19]	Quality of economic evaluations and variability of assumptions of hepatitis B recombinant vaccines	3·75	CBA, CEA, CMA, CUA, unknown (33)	1987–95	Twenty-eight-item checklist; six definitions for study design classification	Main problems are the estimates of incidence of the target disease, estimates of effect of vaccines and variability of methods of evaluation
Diener 1998[20]	Quality of CV methods in economic evaluations	3·93	CCA and CBA (48)	1984–89 and 1990–96	Five-point classification and evaluation checklist based on previous work	Increase in numbers and poor relationship with conceptual framework
Evers 1997[21]	Quality of economic evaluations of mental health care interventions	2·31	CBA, CUA, CEA, CMA and COIs (91)	1971–95	Twenty-one-item checklist	Few good quality economic evaluations were found
Gerard 1992[12]	Quality of CUAs	4·0	CUA (51)	1980–91	Two-stage checklist based on "good practice" principles	Improvements in reporting and evaluations urgently required

Continued

Appendix 6.1 (Continued)

Study (first author and year)	Topic and study question	Mean quality score	Design (number) of included economic evaluations	Year of publication/ preparation of included economic evaluations	Instrument used to assess quality of primary studies	Main study conclusions
Gerard 2000[13]	Quality of CUAs and validation of *BMJ* checklist as quality instrument	4·0	CUA (43)	1996	Thirty-three-item *BMJ* checklist modified for CUA assessment	Over 50% of CUAs included in the review were of unsatisfactory quality
Hill 2000[11]	Description of problems with pharmacoeconomic submissions to Australian Pharmaceutical Benefits Scheme	3·75	Submissions and re-submissions (326)	1994–97	Detailed scrutiny by assessors and committees, re-run of computer models submitted	Two hundred and eighteen submissions (67%) had one or more serious methodological problems
Hutton 1999[22]	Quality of economic evaluations of pneumococcus vaccination in USA	4·0	CBA, CUA, CEA (5)	1980–97	*BMJ* checklist	Considerable variability in methods and underlying assumptions of epidemiology of target disease and effect of vaccines
Jacobs 1998[23]	Quality of indirect cost estimation in economic evaluations	3·25	CEA, CUA and CMA (25)	1994–96	Four-item checklist	Wide variation in methods used
Jefferson 1994[24]	Quality of economic evaluations of HB vaccines	3·75	Economic studies of different design (90)	1982–93	Nineteen-item checklist; five definitions for study design classification	Wide variations in methods used. Epidemiological assumptions of doubtful credibility were used
Jefferson 1996[25]	Quality of economic evaluations of influenza vaccination as a preliminary for defining a secondary model	3·62	Economic studies of different design (31)	1974–94	Six-item checklist	Seventeen studies failed the screening phase, only two because of methodological weaknesses. Considerable variability in underlying assumptions of effect of vaccines

Continued

Appendix 6.1 (Continued)

Study (first author and year)	Topic and study question	Mean quality score	Design (number) of included economic evaluations	Year of publication/ preparation of included economic evaluations	Instrument used to assess quality of primary studies	Main study conclusions
Neumann 2000[14]	Quality of CUA reporting and assessment of changes over time	3·93	CUA (228)	1976–97	Seven-item reporting quality checklist	Variability of reporting methods, with a slight improvement over time. Specialist journals fare worse
Petrou 2000[26]	Quality of economic evaluations of antenatal screening	4·0	Economic evaluations of different design (41)	1991–99	*BMJ* checklist	Poor methodological quality of majority of evaluations. Very narrow definition of benefits adopted by most evaluations
Schrappe 1998[27]	Quality of economic evaluations of public health interventions for HIV prevention in developed countries	3·81	CBA, CEA, CUA (40)	1987–97	*BMJ* checklist	Variability of quality methods. Eleven evaluations did not pose a clear study question and were of poor quality
Späth 1999[28]	Quality of economic evaluation of adjuvant therapy for breast cancer as a preliminary to transfer of data to French health care system	3·75	Economic evaluations of different design (26)	1982–96	Four-point checklist	Seventy-seven percent (20) of evaluations failed the first assessment. Data from the remaining six could not be used due to lack of clarity of reporting. Standardisation of reporting and better methods are needed
Udvarhelyi 1992[29]	Quality of economic evaluations and its variation over two periods	3·87	CBA, CUA, CEA (77 and 46)	1978–80 and 1985–87	Six-point checklist	No significant difference in quality between the two periods. Better reporting of analytical methods in general medical journals

CCA = cost-consequence analysis; CMA = cost-minimisation analysis; CEA = cost-effectiveness analysis; CUA = cost-utility analysis; CBA = cost-benefit analysis; COIs = cost-of-illness studies; RCTs = randomised controlled trials; HSM = health status measures; CV = contingent valuation.

Appendix 6.2 Comparison of quality assessment criteria used in each methodological review with those in the *BMJ* checklist.

Study (first author and year)	Checklist items 1	2	3	4	5	6	7	8	9	10	11	12
Adams 1992[16]	No	No	Yes	Yes	Yes	Yes	No	Yes	Yes	NA	Yes	Yes
Anonymous unpublished[17]	Yes	Yes	Yes	No	No	Yes	No	No	No	No	Yes	Yes
Barber 1998[18]	NA	NA	NA	NA	NA	No	NA	Yes	NA	NA	NA	NA
Brazier 1999[10]	No	No	No	No	No	No	NA	Yes	Yes	NA	Yes	Yes
Demicheli 1997[19]	Yes	Yes	Yes	Yes	Yes	Yes	Yes	Yes	Yes	No	Yes	No
Diener 1998[20]	Yes	No	Yes	No	No	Yes	NA	Yes	Yes	NA	Yes	Yes
Evers 1997[21]	No	No	Yes	No	No	Yes	No	Yes	Yes	Yes	No	Yes
Gerard 1992[12]	Yes	Yes	Yes	Yes	Yes	Yes	Yes	Yes	Yes	Yes	Yes	Yes
Gerard 2000[13]	Yes	Yes	Yes	Yes	Yes	NA	Yes	Yes	NC	NC	Yes	Yes
Hill 2000[11]	Yes	Yes	Yes	Yes	Yes	Yes	NC	Yes	Yes	Yes	Yes	Yes
Hutton 1999[22]	Yes	Yes	Yes	Yes	Yes	Yes	Yes	Yes	Yes	Yes	Yes	Yes
Jacobs 1998[23]	NA	NA	NA	NA	NA	NA	NA	NA	NA	NA	NA	NA
Jefferson 1994[24]	Yes	NA	No	Yes	Yes	Yes	No	Yes	Yes	Yes	Yes	NC
Jefferson 1996[25]	Yes	Yes	Yes	Yes	Yes	NC	NC	NC	NC	NC	NC	NC
Neumann 2000[14]	No	No	Yes	No	Yes	NA	No	Yes	No	No	Yes	Yes
Petrou 2000[26]	Yes	Yes	Yes	Yes	Yes	Yes	Yes	Yes	Yes	Yes	Yes	Yes
Schrappe 1998[27]	Yes	Yes	Yes	Yes	Yes	Yes	Yes	Yes	Yes	Yes	Yes	Yes
Späth 1999[28]	NC	NC	Yes	NC	Yes	Yes	No	No	Yes	Yes	NC	Yes
Udvarhelyi 1992[29]	No	No	Yes	No	No	No	No	No	No	No	Yes	No

Based on the 35 criteria from the *BMJ* guidelines (listed below). Responses to each question can be Yes (covers same criterion as the *BMJ* checklist), No (does not cover this area), NC = not clear. NA = not applicable (to the issues addressed by the included review).

1 Research question stated
2 Importance of question stated
3 Viewpoint of analysis stated and defined
4 Rationale for choosing alternative programmes or interventions compared stated
5 Alternatives being compared clearly defined
6 Form of economic evaluation used stated
7 Choice of form of economic evaluation justified in relation to question addressed
8 Source(s) of effectiveness estimates stated
9 Details of design and results of effectiveness study given (if based on single study)
10 Details of methods of synthesis or meta-analysis of estimates given (if based on overview of a number of effectiveness studies)
11 Primary outcome measure(s) for economic evaluation clearly stated
12 Methods to value health states and other benefits stated

Continued

Appendix 6.2 (Continued)

Study (first author and year)	Checklist items 13	14	15	16	17	18	19	20	21	22	23	24
Adams 1992[16]	Yes	Yes	Yes	No	Yes	Yes	Yes	Yes	Yes	Yes	Yes	NC
Anonymous unpublished[17]	Yes	No	No	No	No	No	No	No	No	No	No	No
Barber 1998[18]	NA	NA	NA	NA	Yes	NA	NA	NA	NA	NA	NA	NA
Brazier 1999[10]	Yes	NA	NA	NA	NA	NA	NA	NA	NA	NA	NA	NA
Demicheli 1997[19]	No	No	No	Yes	Yes	No	No	No	No	Yes	Yes	No
Diener 1998[20]	Yes	NA	NA	NA	NA	NC	NA	No	Yes	NA	NA	NA
Evers 1997[21]	Yes	No	No	Yes	NC	Yes	Yes	No	No	Yes	No	No
Gerard 1992[12]	Yes	Yes	Yes	Yes	Yes	Yes	Yes	No	No	Yes	Yes	No
Gerard 2000[13]	Yes	Yes	Yes	Yes	Yes	Yes	Yes	Yes	Yes	Yes	Yes	Yes
Hill 2000[11]	Yes	NC	NC	NC	NC	Yes	NA	Yes	Yes	Yes	Yes	Yes
Hutton 1999[22]	Yes	Yes	Yes	Yes	Yes	Yes	Yes	Yes	Yes	Yes	Yes	Yes
Jacobs 1998[23]	NA	Yes	Yes	Yes	Yes	Yes	NC	Yes	Yes	Yes	NC	NC
Jefferson 1994[24]	No	Yes	Yes	No	No	Yes	NC	Yes	No	Yes	Yes	No
Jefferson 1996[25]	NC	Yes	NC	Yes	Yes	NC	NC	NC	NC	Yes	NC	NC
Neumann 2000[14]	Yes	NC	NC	No	No	Yes	Yes	Yes	Yes	No	Yes	No
Petrou 2000[26]	Yes	Yes	Yes	Yes	Yes	Yes	Yes	Yes	Yes	Yes	Yes	Yes
Schrappe 1998[27]	Yes	Yes	Yes	Yes	Yes	Yes	Yes	Yes	Yes	Yes	Yes	Yes
Späth 1999[28]	Yes	Yes	Yes	Yes	Yes	NC	NC	Yes	NC	NC	Yes	NC
Udvarhelyi 1992[29]	No	No	NA	No	No	NC	No	No	No	Yes	Yes	No

Based on the 35 criteria from the *BMJ* guidelines (listed below). Responses to each question can be Yes (covers same criterion as the *BMJ* checklist), No (does not cover this area), NC = not clear. NA = not applicable (to the issues addressed by the included review)

13 Details of subjects from whom valuations were obtained given
14 Productivity changes (if included) reported separately
15 Relevance of productivity changes to study question discussed
16 Quantities of resources reported separately from their unit costs
17 Methods for estimation of quantities and unit costs described
18 Currency and price data recorded
19 Details of currency and price adjustments for inflation or currency conversion given
20 Details of any model used
21 Choice of model used and key parameters on which it is based justified
22 Time horizon of costs and benefits stated
23 Discount rate(s) stated
24 Choice of rate(s) justified

Continued

Appendix 6.2 (Continued)

Study (first author and year)	Checklist items 25	26	27	28	29	30	31	32	33	34	35
Adams 1992[16]	NC	No	Yes	Yes	No	Yes	Yes	No	NC	NC	Yes
Anonymous unpublished[17]	No	No	No	No	No	NC	No	No	Yes	Yes	Yes
Barber 1998[18]	NA	Yes	Yes	No	No	NA	NA	No	Yes	Yes	Yes
Brazier 1999[10]	NA	NA	NA	No	NA	NA	NA	NA	NA	NA	NA
Demicheli 1997[19]	Yes	No	Yes	No	Yes	Yes	Yes	No	Yes	Yes	Yes
Diener 1998[20]	No	NA	NA	NA	NA	NA	NA	NA	NA	NA	NA
Evers 1997[21]	No	NC	Yes	No	No	No	Yes	NC	No	No	No
Gerard 1992[12]	NC	No	Yes	No	No	Yes	Yes	—	Yes	Yes	Yes
Gerard 2000[13]	Yes	Yes	Yes	Yes	Yes	Yes	Yes	Yes	Yes	Yes	Yes
Hill 2000[11]	NC	Yes	NC	NC	NC	Yes	Yes	Yes	Yes	Yes	Yes
Hutton 1999[22]	Yes	Yes	Yes	Yes	Yes	Yes	Yes	Yes	Yes	Yes	Yes
Jacobs 1998[23]	NC	No	Yes	No	No	No	NA	NA	Yes	Yes	Yes
Jefferson 1994[24]	No	No	Yes	Yes	No	No	Yes	Yes	Yes	Yes	Yes
Jefferson 1996[25]	NC	Yes	Yes	NC	No	Yes	Yes	No	No	No	No
Neumann 2000[14]	No	No	Yes	No	No	No	Yes	No	NC	Yes	Yes
Petrou 2000[26]	Yes	Yes	Yes	Yes	Yes	Yes	Yes	Yes	Yes	Yes	Yes
Schrappe 1998[27]	Yes	Yes	Yes	Yes	Yes	Yes	Yes	Yes	Yes	Yes	Yes
Späth 1999[28]	NC	NC	No	No	NC	Yes	No	No	No	No	No
Udvarhelyi 1992[29]	No	No	Yes	No	No	No	Yes	No	No	No	No

Based on the 35 criteria from the *BMJ* guidelines (listed below). Responses to each question can be Yes (covers same criterion as the *BMJ* checklist), No (does not cover this area), NC = not clear. NA = not applicable (to the issues addressed by the included review)

25 Explanation given if costs and benefits are not discounted
26 Details of statistical tests and CI given for stochastic data
27 Approach to sensitivity analysis given
28 Choice of variable for sensitivity analysis justified
29 Ranges of which variables are varied stated
30 Relevant alternatives compared
31 Incremental analysis reported
32 Major outcomes presented in an aggregated as well as a disaggregated form
33 Answer to study question given
34 Conclusions follow from data reported
35 Conclusions accompanied by appropriate caveats

Appendix 6.3 Issues relating to the quality of economic evaluations assessed by the included reviews. Part 1: study design, assessment of benefits and assessment of costs.

Study (first author and year)	Study design	Assessment of effectiveness/benefits	Assessment of resource use and costs
Adams 1992[16]	Of the 51 studies that were quality assessed out of a sample of 121 identified 76·5% were CEA, 15·7% CBA; with the remainder the type of evaluation was unclear. Only a quarter of studies reported perspective, other measures to assess quality of study type not reported or assessed	74·5% of studies were prospectively designed but appropriate measures of benefits and cost were only recorded in 23·5%	Studies assessed on appropriateness of costs and benefits, separate information on the quality of costs measurement was not reported in this review
Anonymous unpublished[17]	Of the 87 studies identified 62·1% were CEA, 17·2% were CBA, 13·8% CMA and 5·9% were CUAs. The objective of the studies did not appear to be linked to a policy decision in 73·6% of cases. The perspective was not stated in 72·4% of studies	The majority of studies (67·2%) obtained data from the literature. Of the 6 CUAs only 2 reported explicit designs. However both of these used a discredited valuation (Rosser matrix)	18·4% of studies included indirect costs as well as direct costs. The sources of cost data were not reported in 24·1% of studies
Barber 1998[18]	Not applicable to topic of review	Not applicable to topic of review	Collection of costs not main topic for the review
Brazier 1999[10]	Not applicable to topic of review	285 papers were identified which looked at a spectrum of health status measures. These measures were assessed against 5 criteria: practicality, reliability, descriptive validity, valuation and empirical validity. None of the methods appeared dominant over these criteria. The best-preference-based measures appeared to be the EQ-5D of health utilities index	Not applicable to topic of review
Demicheli 1997[19]	33 studies were identified of which 45·5% took a societal viewpoint, 39·4% the health care system; 11 studies were reported by their authors as being CBA, 16 reported as CEA, 1 as CMA and 2 as CUA. In 2 cases the type of design was unclear. However in 11 studies the stated design was incorrect.	Outcome measures varied markedly between studies	57·5% reported how costs were derived but only 21·2% reported resource use and unit costs

Continued

Appendix 6.3 (Continued)

Study (first author and year)	Study design	Assessment of effectiveness/benefits	Assessment of resource use and costs
Diener 1998[20]	Of the 48 studies identified over 80% stated they were CBA; very few actually were. Other aspects of study design were not assessed	Many different methods of contingent valuation were used but methods were not well reported	Not applicable to topic of review
Evers 1997[21]	Report of perspective was poor with 6·5% of 91 studies explicitly mentioning it. Difficult to make judgements as to whether design was correctly defined or appropriate to the question aspects of quality were not reported	Only 30% of the studies had a randomised or quasi-randomised design and therefore the basis of study design would not control for biases in the majority of cases. Methods of valuation of health states was varied	Relatively few studies (9%) measured indirect costs and methods were often unclear. Methods of cost measurement often poor with reliance of charges (all except 4 studies) without consideration of whether these represented opportunity costs opportunity costs
Gerard 1992[12]	Baseline comparisons were often poorly defined and in 6% of the 51 studies it was not possible to judge what the comparator was. The majority (92%) of studies stated a perspective. 27·5% of studies were conducted as CUAs but could have been undertaken as CEAs	The source of effectiveness data was clearly described in 59% of studies but may not have adequately controlled biases in at least 63% of studies. Focus of QALY valuation focused more on quality rather than length of life. Source of valuations was omitted in 27% of studies and was definitely inappropriate in 8%. Many different measures were used and in at least 10% of studies insufficient information was available to determine the method	The majority of studies presented only direct costs (88%). In 27·5% of studies it was unclear whether the appropriate costs were identified and measured. Furthermore, inadequate description was provided in 40% of studies about how costs were valued. 22% of studies did not give an explicit price base
Gerard 2000[13]	The viewpoint of the analysis was not adequately justified in 81% of the 43 identified studies	The source of data used as the basis of health state valuations was not considered but in 51% of cases inadequate description of methods of QALY estimation were given, including a similar proportion that failed to provide sufficient details of who provided valuations	Unit costs were not adequately reported separately in 86% of studies and the methods used to estimate resource use were not adequately explained in 58% of studies
Hill 2000[11]	Of the 326 studies many of these aspects of quality were determined by the purpose the evaluation was required for. However, the choice of comparator was in dispute in 6% of cases	Studies were shown to use poor quality data (12·4%), 13% suffered problems in analysis of the data, 6% used inappropriate outcomes and 6% failed to use the relevant existing data. Studies using WTP or QALYs have used inappropriate questionnaires or sample sizes	Analysis of costs often lacked transparency and in 13% of cases there were problems in calculation of costs

Continued

Appendix 6.3 (Continued)

Study (first author and year)	Study design	Assessment of effectiveness/benefits	Assessment of resource use and costs
Hutton 1999[22]	In an assessment of 5 evaluations of pneumococcal vaccines 3 were CUA, 1 CBA and 1 CEA. The study question was always clearly stated and the alternatives were clearly described. However they were rarely justified	There was a general failure to give details of the studies from which effectiveness data were drawn	There was inconsistency in the treatment of indirect costs and a failure to report resource use and costs separately
Jacobs 1998[23]	Not applicable to topic of review	Not applicable to topic of review	Focus was solely on indirect costs. In all but 12% of the 25 studies it is unclear whether the time horizon was appropriate to estimate indirect costs. 12% of studies included indirect costs falling on patients and care-givers. There was a great deal of variability in terms of what aspects of activity were included in indirect costs and how they were valued
Jefferson 1994[24]	All studies provided a clearly defined study question. The stated design and the actual design did not agree in 38% of cases	Sources of data were defined. But the time span used to estimate costs may have been too short. 12% of studies did not include health outcome measures and relied solely on human capital	No study covered all the areas of costs that may be considered relevant. The time span used to estimate costs may have been too short in some studies
Jefferson 1996[25]	31 studies were identified of which 14 were finally included. Only 2 were excluded due to methodological problems	These aspects were not reported in the review	These aspects were not reported in the review
Neumann 2000[14]	The study perspective was stated in approximately 50% of 228 studies included. This percentage remained fairly constant over time. The comparator used in the study was adequately described in over 80% of cases but may have slightly decreased over time	The reporting of methods of eliciting preferences and the source of valuations was nearly always over 75% but appeared to have deteriorated over time	The estimation of net costs and the source of unit costs were reported in over 80% of cases and if anything seemed to improve. The price base was less well reported (maximum of 70% of cases) and did not differ over time

Continued

Appendix 6.3 (Continued)

Study (first author and year)	Study design	Assessment of effectiveness/benefits	Assessment of resource use and costs
Petrou 2000[26]	Only 9 of the 41 studies adopted a societal perspective	Modelling methods were used in the majority of studies. The outcome measures chosen would not have captured all relevant benefits in 7 studies. A further 17 on examination proved to be cost-analyses only	9 studies considered indirect costs and other non-health care costs. Diaggregated cost data was rarely reported and it is likely that at least 6 studies failed to include significant items of cost
Schrappe 2000[27]	Of the 40 studies identified 22 were CEA, 15 CBA and 3 CUA. However, this was only explicitly stated in 75%. The research question was not stated in 37·5%. The majority of studies reported data from the societal perspective (85%)	In 95% of cases the source of data was stated. The most common outcome was diagnosis of HIV (27·5%). Varying definitions of transmission were used in 20%. Lives saved or life years were used in 12·5% and QALYs in 7·5%	82·5% described the estimation of resources and unit costs but only 27% reported them separately. Indirect costs were included in 52·5% but they were not reported separately in 7·5% of studies
Späth 1999[28]	34 studies were identified of which 3% were rejected as the perspective could not be identified, they were cost analyses (31%), didn't involve a comparison (54%), no description of alternative (4%) or the comparator was not relevant (15%). 4 of the remaining studies were CUA, 1 was CEA and 1 CMA	3 were based on decision analysis and 3 on clinical trials	Direct medical costs were included in all but no other costs. Description of cost methodology and reporting of costs was poor in all studies
Udvarhelyi 1992[29]	Only 18% reported the perspective	The nature of benefit assessed (if any) was unclear in 17% of studies	4% of studies failed to provide an estimate of costs at all. Only 4% included all components of cost and only few considered costs of adverse effects/morbidity or costs averted

CEA = cost-effectiveness analysis; CBA = cost-benefit analysis; CMA = cost-minimisation analysis; CUA = cost-utility analysis; QALY = quality-adjusted life year; RCT = randomised controlled trial; WTP = willingness to pay.

Appendix 6.4 Issues relating to the quality of economic evaluations assessed by the included reviews. Part 2: analysis and conclusions.

Study (first author and year)	Methods of analysis	Discussion and conclusions
Adams 1992[16]	Quality of analysis not reported except that in less than 16% of studies was sensitivity analysis of costs performed and less than 8% on benefits. Incremental analysis was rarely consistent with the perspective	Distributional effects of the alternatives were not considered by over 50% of the studies
Anonymous unpublished[17]	28·7% of studies used decision analytic techniques. No other aspects of quality were reported	62·1% of studies made recommendations for decision making although most did not have objectives linked to a specific policy decision (73·6%)
Barber 1998[18]	45 papers were identified and major deficiencies were found in the way cost data derived from RCTs are analysed. Only 20% reported adequate measures of variability. 56% reported statistical tests between groups. Sensitivity analysis rarely performed. Issues such as missing data (details of completeness given in 53%), sample sizes (provided in only 16% of studies and never for economic outcomes) inadequately addressed	Conclusions based on results were not justified in 64% of cases
Brazier 1999[10]	Not applicable to topic of review	Not applicable to topic of review
Demicheli 1997[19]	Only 57·5% stated information on time span of the analysis and only 45·5% performed discounting. Incremental analysis was mentioned or performed in 21·2% of studies. Sensitivity analysis was performed in 54·5% (18) of studies but this was limited to one-way analysis in 10 studies. 17 studies used threshold analysis and one used probabilistic sensitivity analysis	Outcomes that were favourable to the programme of vaccination were reported in 66·6% of the studies but these conclusions were never warranted by the evidence
Diener 1998[20]	Not applicable to topic of review	These issues were not covered by the review
Evers 1997[21]	Incremental analysis rarely performed (6% of studies), 40% used discounting appropriately and reported costs in a base year. Only 10% of studies performed sensitivity analysis (whether such analysis was appropriate was not assessed)	These issues were not covered by the review

Continued

Appendix 6.4 (Continued)

Study (first author and year)	Methods of analysis	Discussion and conclusions
Gerard 1992[12]	27% of studies looked at average costs only, however it was unclear whether they provided a suitable proxy for marginal costs. Similarly for those studies that looked at marginal cost it was unclear whether they had looked at the correct margin as the scale of the change was not often stated. 71% of studies used appropriate discounting but only 37% provided extensive sensitivity analysis	Caveats particularly in the use of health state valuations were rarely made. The results were often placed in context in league tables, which in some cases could be seriously misleading
Gerard 2000[13]	Choice of discount rate was fully justified in 15% of studies and no study that did not discount cost and benefits provided a full explanation for not discounting. The justification of the choice of variables and the extent to which they were varied and extent of sensitivity analysis was not fully given in 72% and 74% of studies. 7% of studies did not appear to conduct any sensitivity analysis	Almost all studies failed to put their results in context by comparison with results from other studies that used similar methods and were conducted in a similar setting. Other aspects of quality not otherwise specifically mentioned had been fully addressed in over 50% of the studies
Hill 2000[11]	Problems were found relating to discounting, relating costs to outcomes and handling uncertainties associated with the extrapolation of results (9·6%). Several studies also contained basic analysis errors (4%). Modelling assumptions were not justified in 4% of studies	Problems identified with analyses had the potential to distort conclusions and change recommendations. Many of the problems only became apparent because of the nature of the information available to the reviewers
Hutton 1999[22]	Although discounting was always appropriately performed the rates were rarely justified and there was an extremely wide variation in time horizons. Sensitivity analysis was always performed but again rarely justified	These issues were not covered by the review
Jacobs 1998[23]	No study performed adequate sensitivity analysis around the magnitude of direct costs. Inclusion/exclusion of indirect costs was shown to significantly affect the conclusions of a study	Not applicable to topic of review
Jefferson 1994[24]	A variety of analytic approaches was used including Markov models. 24·4% clearly gave the discount rate and in half of these a rationale for the use of this rate was given. Univariant or multivarient sensitivity analysis was performed in 41% of cases. Only 9% of studies used marginal cost estimates	All studies reached conclusions but only for a few were these valid because of uncertain or unclear methodology. Only 10% of studies fulfilled a minimum quality checklist although one criterion was that costs should be reported in US$ to aid comparability
Jefferson 1996[25]	These aspects were not reported in the review	These aspects not reported in the review

Continued

Appendix 6.4 (Continued)

Study (first author and year)	Methods of analysis	Discussion and conclusions
Neumann 2000[14]	When modelling was performed its assumptions and description were provided in 82·5% and 53·5% of studies. Reporting appeared to improve over time. Discounting was performed in 64·9% of studies and appeared to be less frequently performed in later studies. Incremental analysis was performed in 46% of studies overall and its use increased over time. Sensitivity analysis was performed in 89% of studies overall and its use appeared to be increasing over time. Sensitivity analysis was less frequently performed on specific aspects, for example, costs and preferences, but its use generally increased over time	The limitations of conclusions were discussed in 84% of studies overall and this discussion increased over time. However the ethical implications were discussed in only 27% of studies overall and this type of discussion declined over time
Petrou 2000[26]	Three studies failed to discount future costs. Sensitivity analysis was either not used at all or in 10 studies applied to clinical or epidemiological parameters only	These aspects were not reported in the review
Schrappe 1998[27]	Incremental analysis was performed in 52·5% of studies but corrections for inflation were only given in 2 of 30 cases where it was relevant and the year of cost data was given in 60%. Discounting was not appropriately performed in 6 of the 29 studies where it was required. Sensitivity analysis was performed in only 58% of studies	These aspects were not reported in the review
Späth 1999[28]	These aspects were not reported in the review	The study's results were not eligible for transfer to the French health care system
Udvarhelyi 1992[29]	48% of studies appropriately used discounting and only 305 of studies used sensitivity analysis. Incremental analysis was used in 25% of cases	These issues were not covered by this review

RCTs = randomised controlled trials; CUA = cost-utility analysis; CCA = cost-consequence analysis.

References

1 Elixhauser A. Health care cost-benefit analysis and cost-effectiveness analysis. From 1979 to 1990: a bibliography. *Med Care* 1993;**31**:JS1–150.
2 Elixhauser A, Halpern M, Schmier J, Luce BR. Health care CBA and CEA from 1991 to 1996: an updated bibliography. *Med Care* 1998;**36**:MS1–147.
3 Drummond M, Jefferson T and the BMJ Economic Evaluation Working Party. Guidelines for authors and peer reviewers of economic submissions to the BMJ. The BMJ Economic Evaluation Working Party. *BMJ* 1996;**313**:275–83.
4 Jefferson T, Demicheli V. Are guidelines for peer-reviewing economic evaluations necessary? A survey of current editorial practice. *Health Econ* 1995;**4**:383–8.
5 Demicheli V, Hutton J. Peer review of economic submissions. In: Godlee F, Jefferson T, eds. *Peer review in health science*. London: BMJ Books, 1999.
6 Jefferson TO, Demicheli V, Vale L. The quality of systematic reviews of economic evaluations in healthcare and what they are telling us: it is time for action. Presented at the 4th International Congress of Peer Review, Barcelona, September 2001.
7 Oxman AD, Guyatt GH. Validation of an index of the quality of review articles. *J Clin Epidemiol* 1991;**44**:1271–8.
8 Oxman AD, Cook DJ, Guyatt GH. Users' guides to the medical literature. VI. How to use an overview. Evidence-Based Medicine Working Group. *JAMA* 1994;**272**:1367–71.
9 Mulrow CD, Cook DJ. *Systematic reviews: synthesis of best evidence for healthcare*. Philadelphia: American College of Physicians, 1998.
10 Brazier J, Deverill M, Green C, Harper R, Booth A. A review of the use of health status measures in economic evaluation. *Health Technol Assess* 1999;**3**:i–164.
11 Hill SR, Mitchell AS, Henry DA. Problems with the interpretation of pharmacoeconomic analyses: a review of submissions to the Australian Pharmaceutical Benefits Scheme. *JAMA* 2000;**283**:2116–21.
12 Gerard K. Cost-utility in practice: a policy maker's guide to the state of the art. *Health Policy* 1992;**21**:249–79.
13 Gerard K, Seymour J, Smoker I. A tool to improve quality of reporting published economic analyses. *Int J Technol Assess Health Care* 2000;**16**:100–10.
14 Neumann PJ, Stone PW, Chapman RH, Sandberg EA, Bell CM. The quality of reporting in published cost-utility analyses, 1976-1997. *Ann Intern Med* 2000;**132**:964–72.
15 Briggs AH, Gray AM. Handling uncertainty when performing economic evaluation of healthcare interventions. *Health Technol Assess* 1999;**3**:1–134.
16 Adams M, McCall N, Gray D, Orza M, Chalmers TC. Economic analysis in randomised controlled trials. *Med Care* 1992;**30**:231–8.
17 Anonymous. Twenty years of health care economic evaluations in Spain: are we doing well? Unpublished work, 2001.
18 Barber JA, Thompson SG. Analysis and interpretation of cost data in randomised controlled trials: review of published studies. *BMJ* 1998;**317**:1195–200.
19 Demicheli V, Jefferson T. An exploratory review of the economics of recombinant vaccines against hepatitis B (HB). In: Ronchi E, ed. *The economic aspect of biotechnologies related to human health: biotechnology and medical innovation: socio-economic assessment of the technology, the potential and the products*. Paris: OECD, 1997.
20 Diener A, O'Brien B, Gafni A. Health care contingent valuation studies: a review and classification of the literature. *Health Econ* 1998;**7**:313–26.
21 Evers SM, Van Wijk AS, Ament AJ. Economic evaluation of mental health care interventions. A review. *Health Econ* 1997;**6**:161–77.
22 Hutton J, Iglesias C, Jefferson TO. Assessing the potential cost effectiveness of pneumococcal vaccines in the US: methodological issues and current evidence. *Drugs Aging* 1999;**15** (Suppl 1):31–6.
23 Jacobs P, Fassbender K. The measurement of indirect costs in the health economics evaluation literature. A review. *Int J Technol Assess Health Care* 1998;**14**:799–808.
24 Jefferson T, Demicheli V. Is vaccination against hepatitis B efficient? A review of world literature. *Health Econ* 1994;**3**:25–37.
25 Jefferson T, Demicheli V. Economic evaluation of influenza vaccination and economic modelling. Can results be pooled? *Pharmacoeconomics* 1996;**9** (Suppl 3):67–72.
26 Petrou S, Henderson J, Roberts T, Martin MA. Recent economic evaluations of antenatal screening: a systematic review and critique. *J Med Screen* 2000;**7**:59–73.

27 Schrappe M, Lauterbach K. Systematic review on the cost-effectiveness of public health interventions for HIV prevention in industrialized countries. *AIDS* 1998;**12** (Suppl A): S231–8.

28 Späth HM, Carrere MO, Fervers B, Philip T. Analysis of the eligibility of published economic evaluations for transfer to a given health care system. Methodological approach and application to the French health care system. *Health Policy* 1999;**49**:161–77.

29 Udvarhelyi IS, Colditz GA, Rai A, Epstein AM. Cost-effectiveness and cost-benefit analyses in the medical literature. Are the methods being used correctly? *Ann Intern Med* 1992;**116**:238–44.

7: Effectiveness estimates in economic evaluation

VITTORIO DEMICHELI, TOM JEFFERSON, LUKE VALE

Introduction

Economic evaluation has become globally established as a crucial support for decision making in health care.[1] Its rise in popularity is reflected by the increasing number of published studies of all designs.[2,3] Although the availability of results of economic evaluations is increasing, as is the willingness to use them to aid allocation of scarce health care resources, there is the need for policy decisions made on the basis of published studies to be ethically sound and not misled by poor quality. As reported in Chapter 6, in the early 1990s several systematic reviews of economic studies cast doubt on the scientific reliability of a proportion of published evaluations. All advocated better standards of conducting and reporting economic evaluations.[4–7]

In this chapter the evidence of effectiveness that was used in a sample of published economic evaluations is identified and assessed. Consideration is then given to whether estimates of effectiveness derived from systematic reviews that existed prior to the publication of the economic evaluations themselves could possibly have been incorporated in the evaluations. Finally, a case study is presented to illustrate the likely effect of incorporating poor economic methodology in randomised controlled trials (RCTs) evaluating the effectiveness of a complex intervention.

Background

As Jefferson *et al* reported in Chapter 6, a review of the quality of unpublished economic evaluations of 326 pharmacoeconomic submissions made between 1994 and 1997 by industry to the Australian reimbursement authority provides a glimpse of the nature and the extent of the main methodological problems. Two hundred and eighteen submissions (67% of the total) showed major methodological problems, with 31 of these showing more than one. Sixty-two per cent of problems related to the choice of estimates for effectiveness of the evaluated pharmaceuticals and 28·5% to methods of modelling and related clinical assumptions.[8] Methodological problems were found to be widespread when reviewing the results of systematic reviews of economic evaluations.[9] The use of reliable effectiveness estimates in economic evaluations to assess the likely impact of the intervention under scrutiny is one of the key methodological aspects present in the various recommendations issued.[10,11]

Clinical trials are regarded as the most powerful tool to assess the effectiveness of interventions and economic analysis should be based on their results. Therefore, one of the reasons advocated for the routine introduction of economic analysis alongside clinical trials is the need to base the evaluation on reliable estimates of effectiveness.[12]

Systematic reviews of RCTs (and of other study designs where RCTs have not been performed or may not be possible or appropriate) are likely to provide more reliable information on relative effectiveness than other sources of evidence on the differential effects of alternative forms of health care.[13] When available, effectiveness estimates from systematic reviews of RCTs should be preferentially used in any form of economic evaluation of health care interventions. Previous reviews and anecdotal evidence would seem to suggest that few estimates from systematic reviews are actually incorporated into economic evaluations.

Methods

Identification of economic evaluations that used systematically derived evidence on effectiveness

Economic evaluations on different topics were identified from the NHS Economic Evaluation Database (NHS EED, NHS Centre for Reviews and Dissemination, University of York, 2001). The choice of topics was determined on the basis of the existence of specific Cochrane Review Groups with a high number of systematic reviews published in the Cochrane Library, Issue 2, 2001. Ten topics were identified (communicable disease, hypertension, menstrual disorders, musculoskeletal disease, neonatal diseases, pregnancy and childbirth, schizophrenia, stroke, vaccines and wound infections). The identification of studies was carried out applying the relevant MeSH terms covering each area as specified in the Thesaurus of the Cochrane Library.

From the abstract of each study the following pieces of information were extracted:

1 Study design as assessed by the NHS EED. When more than one study design was present in the same paper, the more complex one was recorded. Cost-benefit analysis (CBA) was considered to be more complex than cost-utility analysis (CUA) and CUA more complex than cost-effectiveness analysis (CEA).

2 The types of effectiveness estimates used in the economic evaluations, as reported by NHS EED, were classified as follows:

- Authors' or other experts' opinions – when at least one of the estimates of effect was based only on assumptions.
- Single study – when at least one of the estimates of effect was based on the result of a single study regardless of the study design (RCT or other).
- Review – when the estimates of effect were based on the results of more than one study derived from the literature and presented in a descriptive way.
- Systematic review – when the estimates of effect were based on the results of more than one study systematically identified, assessed and synthesised.

Identification of economic evaluations that potentially could have been based on Cochrane reviews

The NHS EED was searched to identify published economic evaluations that could have incorporated the results of completed Cochrane reviews. Each Cochrane review was identified by searching the Cochrane Library with the same MeSH terms used for the topic areas listed above.

The following information was recorded for each identified review:

- Type of intervention or research question.
- Date of first publication of the review in the Cochrane Library.

A review was considered as "usable" as a source of estimates of effectiveness in a published economic evaluation if it addressed the same research question and was published prior to (the year before) the economic evaluation.

Case study: the use of chemotherapy as an intervention for colorectal cancer

To illustrate the likely effect of the incorporation of poor economic methodology in RCTs evaluating the effectiveness of complex intervention, a systematic review of 13 RCTs on chemotherapy of colorectal cancer was used. These studies were assessed on the basis of the methods used to assess quality of life, methods and reporting of resource and cost and finally methods and reporting of relative efficiency.

Results

Identification of economic evaluations that used systematically derived evidence on effectiveness

Table 7.1 shows the number of abstracts identified as being relevant to each topic area and the number of those that were assessed by their design

Table 7.1 Number and type of economic evaluations identified on NHS EED.

	Abstracts identified	Classified as economic evaluation	Type of economic evaluation		
			CEA	CUA	CBA
Communicable disease	15	3	3	0	0
Hypertension	119	35	33	2	0
Menstrual disorders	14	7	6	1	0
Musculoskeletal disease	210	49	40	9	0
Neonatal diseases	173	69	60	5	4
Pregnancy and childbirth	203	102	97	3	2
Schizophrenia	104	17	13	4	0
Stroke	165	61	37	21	3
Vaccines	103	57	49	4	4
Wound infections	40	20	19	1	0

Table 7.2 Sources of evidence on effectiveness for economic evaluations by topic.

	Authors' assumptions	Single study	Literature review	Systematic review
Communicable disease	0	3	0	0
Hypertension	3	19	8	5
Menstrual disorders	1	6	0	0
Musculoskeletal disease	8	28	12	1
Neonatal diseases	10	45	14	0
Pregnancy and childbirth	6	65	22	9
Schizophrenia	2	14	0	1
Stroke	10	26	19	6
Vaccines	18	12	25	2
Wound infections	1	14	5	0
Total	59 **(14%)**	232 **(55%)**	105 **(25%)**	24 **(6%)**

classification as being economic evaluations rather than cost analyses or methodology studies. A total of 1146 abstracts were assessed. Of these, 420 were considered to be economic evaluations, 357 of these being CEAs, 50 CUAs and 13 CBAs. Pregnancy and childbirth accounted for the largest number of economic evaluations (102 out of 203 abstracts assessed). The smallest number of abstracts classified as economic evaluations were related to communicable diseases (3 out of 15 or 20%), whilst the smallest proportion of abstracts classified as economic evaluations relates to schizophrenia (17 out of 104, 16%).

In Table 7.2, the economic evaluations are classified according to the broad categories of effectiveness estimates used in the study. Based on the abstracts reported in the NHS EED the vast majority of economic evaluations identified in this exercise used potentially poor quality effectiveness data. Fifty-five per cent were based on single studies and 14% were based on author(s)' assumptions or expert opinions. Approximately one third of identified economic studies from various topic areas were based upon reviews but only 6% of these were based upon systematic reviews. No information was available about the quality of the reviews or systematic reviews that the identified economic studies used. It is also unclear from the content of the NHS EED whether the economic evaluations identified made attempts to use the best evidence available at the time the study was conducted.

The use of systematic reviews as a source of effectiveness estimates was higher for hypertension. However, four of the five studies that cited systematic reviews as the source of effectiveness estimates referred to the same meta-analysis of studies on the treatment of hypertension.

Identification of economic evaluations that potentially could have been based on Cochrane reviews

Table 7.3 shows the number of systematic reviews published in the Cochrane Library which were "usable" as the source of estimates of effectiveness in published economic evaluations but were not so used.

In the specific field of hypertension, of the 162 complete reviews published only one covered the same research question (the treatment of hypertension in diabetic patients) as one of the economic studies identified and the review was published before the economic study.

Five reviews out of 33 published in the field of musculoskeletal diseases were identified as "usable" as sources of effectiveness estimates by the economic studies; three were on osteoporosis, one on lumbar discectomy and part of one on the treatment of rheumatoid arthritis.

Two systematic reviews were found on the topic of screening for cystic fibrosis (out of the 96 available in the field) which were "usable" as a source of estimates of effectiveness in economic studies.

A total of 167 completed reviews were identified in the field of pregnancy and childbirth. Six published economic evaluations could possibly have

Table 7.3 Number of economic evaluations that could have used Cochrane reviews as a source of effectiveness estimates but failed to do so.

Topic	Completed reviews at March 2001	Published economic evaluations that could have used review findings
Communicable disease	40	0
Hypertension	162	1
Menstrual disorders	46	0
Musculoskeletal disease	33	5
Neonatal diseases	96	2
Pregnancy and childbirth	167	6
Schizophrenia	53	2
Stroke	48	0
Vaccines	35	2
Wound infections	11	0
Colorectal cancer	4	0

used the results of reviews. One study was on early ultrasound scanning; three were on external cephalic version, one on the use of oral zidovudine for the prevention of HIV infection and one on the induction of labour with oxytocin.

For schizophrenia, one review on the effect of olanzapine and haloperidol (out of 53 published) was available before the publication of two economic studies that addressed the same subject.

On the topic of vaccines, only two economic evaluations (on pertussis vaccines and on hepatitis B vaccines in health care workers) of the 35 available were published after the reviews had become available and could have incorporated the results of the review in the analysis. The two economic evaluations were, however, conducted alongside RCTs.

No economic evaluations were identified that could have used completed Cochrane reviews in communicable diseases, menstrual disorders, stroke, cancer care and wound infections.

It should be noted that for some of the economic evaluations mentioned, it is possible that the studies were carried out before the review and only published much later.

Case study: the use of chemotherapy as an intervention for colorectal cancer

The 13 studies were all of randomised or quasi-randomised design, comparing the effects of first or second line chemotherapy with either best available palliative supportive care and/or delayed chemotherapy. Six (46%) of the thirteen studies included in the review contained measures that incorporated a comparative degree of patient well being and satisfaction. However, no two studies used the same complete sets of quality of life (QoL) instruments. Only one study used a colorectal cancer-specific complete QoL instrument (the EORTC QLQ-C30). Four of the six studies used non-cancer-specific instruments and the viewpoint of the evaluation of QoL was mostly unclear. Two of the thirteen (13%) studies produced some evidence of resource consumption and/or of costs per outcome incurred. The usefulness of any economic evidence provided was limited by its poor economic methodology and reporting. For example, resources were not shown separately from unit costs, a finding which echoes that of other systematic reviews.

Discussion

The findings of this research must at this stage remain tentative, but it is clear that a number of economic evaluations have not been based on best available effectiveness data. Even where attempts have been made to base the evaluation on the review of existing research, reviews have not been conducted systematically and their results are likely to be subject to bias in both the selection and synthesis of data. Relatively few published economic evaluations could have used the results of Cochrane reviews instead of the evidence they actually did use. To a certain extent this is not surprising, given the relatively short period of existence of the Cochrane Library and the lack of present coverage of the NHS EED. The former point will limit the possibility that an economic evaluation based on a Cochrane review will have been published and the latter point minimises the possibility of identifying published economic evaluations that could have used such information. Nevertheless, the fact that economic evaluations were identified that had either failed to incorporate estimates of effect from existing systematic reviews or had not used the reviews to set their results in the context of all available evidence, is a cause for concern.

The findings so far indicate a wide range of methodological problems in large parts of the economic literature, especially in the choice of estimates of effect incorporated in economic evaluations. The relationship with decision making is, however, less clear cut as evidence of use of economic evaluations in decision making is not strong.

The potential impact of using weak research evidence to allocate resources is nowhere more evident than in a systematic review of 13 studies of the effects of palliative chemotherapy for advanced colorectal cancer (Colorectal Cancer Collaborative Group, 2000). Two major economic points stand out from this example. First, chemotherapy for colorectal cancer is carried out to improve survival and the quality of remaining life in what is a very harrowing disease for both patients and their families. Although not immediately clear from the text of some of the 13 studies included in the review, these are the universally accepted aims of chemotherapy. The absence of QoL measures in seven of the thirteen RCTs (and the disparate nature of toxicity classification and reporting) is an indictment of the quality of research in this key area. It reveals ignorance of one of the basic rules of research: evaluation of an intervention must be based on its objectives. Even when QoL measures were included, the variety of ad hoc measures developed or used in the studies made any direct comparison impossible. Although some studies were carried out before the development of a complete colorectal cancer-specific measure (the EORTC QLQ-C30), its present availability makes its use in any future studies a sensible step. Second, all studies were carried out in, or focused on, identical settings (oncology units) characterised by high capital and revenue costs. The studies addressed the minimisation of morbidity and mortality for what is now a highly prevalent disease in Western society and the third largest cause of cancer death in the UK and the rest of the developed world. Given the incomplete nature of the evidence presented it is debatable whether any more investment in tertiary care infrastructure should be contemplated until good evidence of effect is available.

Conclusions

The conclusions of this chapter must remain tentative given the relative lack of coverage of the databases used. However, the belief of the authors is that the evidence presented points to major gaps in the conduct and reporting of economic evaluations and among these one of the major areas for improvement is that of the assessment of effectiveness of the interventions evaluated. While it is possible that single RCTs or reviews of RCTs may not have been available at the time of the conduct of the economic evaluation, a significant proportion of evaluations rely on estimates of effect derived from single, small, non-randomised studies or, possibly even worse, expert opinion. This is not an ethically defensible practice if better quality estimates of effect were available at the time the study was conducted. The research community should take urgent steps to rectify or ameliorate the problem.

Summary points

- When available, good quality evidence from systematic reviews of effectiveness should be used in economic evaluation.
- The quality of primary research combined in systematic review is often insufficient to address economic issues.

References

1 Drummond MF, Cooke J, Walley T. Economic evaluation in healthcare decision-making: evidence from the UK. Centre for Health Economics Discussion Paper. University of York, 1996.
2 Elixhauser A. Health care cost-benefit analysis and cost-effectiveness analysis. From 1979 to 1990: a bibliography. *Med Care* 1993;**31**:JS1–150.
3 Elixhauser A, Halpern M, Schmier J, Luce BR. Health care CBA and CEA from 1991 to 1996: an updated bibliography. *Med Care* 1998;**36**:MS1–147.

4 Udvarhelyi IS, Colditz GA, Rai A, Epstein AM. Cost-effectiveness and cost-benefit analyses in the medical literature. Are the methods being used correctly? *Ann Intern Med* 1992;**116**:238–44.
5 Gerard K. Cost-utility in practice: a policy maker's guide to the state of the art. *Health Policy* 1992;**21**:249–79.
6 Adams M, McCall N, Gray D, Orza M, Chalmers TC. Economic analysis in randomised controlled trials. *Med Care* 1992;**30**:231–8.
7 Jefferson T, Demicheli V. Is vaccination against hepatitis B efficient? A review of world literature. *Health Econ* 1994;**3**:25–37.
8 Hill SR, Mitchell AS, Henry DA. Problems with the interpretation of pharmacoeconomic analyses: a review of submissions to the Australian Pharmaceutical Benefits Scheme. *JAMA* 2000;**283**:2116–21.
9 Jefferson TO, Demicheli V. The quality of systematic reviews of economic evaluations in healthcare and what they are telling us: it is time for action. Presented at Fourth International Congress on Peer Review and Global Communication, Barcelona, 2001.
10 Drummond MF, Jefferson TO and the BMJ Economic Evaluation Working Party. Guidelines for authors and peer reviewers of economic submissions to the *BMJ*. *BMJ* 1996;**313**:275–83.
11 Drummond M, Brandt A, Luce B, Rovira J. Standardizing methodologies for economic evaluation in health care. Practice, problems, and potential. *Int J Technol Assess Health Care* 1993;**9**:26–36.
12 Drummond MF. *Economic analysis alongside controlled trials: an introduction for clinical researchers*. London: Department of Health, 1994.
13 Kunz R, Oxman AD. The unpredictability paradox: review of empirical comparisons of randomised and non-randomised clinical trials. *BMJ* 1998;**317**:1185–90.

8: Criteria list for conducting systematic reviews based on economic evaluation studies – the ☑ CHEC project

ANDRE AMENT, SILVIA EVERS, MARIELLE GOOSSENS, HENRICA DE VET, MAURITS VAN TULDER

Introduction

Health care professionals, consumers, researchers and policy makers can be overwhelmed by the sometimes unmanageably large number of studies on the effectiveness and efficiency of health care interventions. Systematic reviews of these studies can help in making well-informed decisions on which intervention to adopt. For maximum usefulness, systematic reviews of economic evaluations should be consistent, of high methodological quality and informative. In this chapter, the ☑ CHEC project is presented;* this project aims to develop a criteria list for systematic reviews of economic evaluations. The criteria list contains a minimum set of items that should be mentioned in every systematic review regarding the methodology of those individual economic evaluations being reviewed. In order to be widely accepted by the scientific community, the list has been developed

* The ☑ CHEC project is a cooperative effort of the Department of Health Organisation Policy and Economics of Maastricht University, the Institute for Rehabilitation Research, Hoensbroek, and the Institute for Research in Extramural Medicine of the Vrije Universiteit Medical Centre, Amsterdam.

collaboratively by an international panel of experts on economic evaluation. Similar calls have been made by others in this volume (see Jefferson *et al*, Chapter 6).

In this chapter, the background of economic evaluations and the need for systematic reviews is described, as well as the importance of guideline development, in this area. Criteria lists are then distinguished from guidelines, before going on to describe the development of a criteria list. Development of the list is described in two further sections – one in which existing guidelines are compared and one in which a Delphi survey is used. Finally, some conclusions are drawn, based on the research so far, and some points for further research are noted.

Background

Economic evaluations are a relatively recent phenomenon. Although some preliminary attempts to assess the benefits of possible health care interventions in economic terms were made in earlier centuries, economic evaluations or medical technology assessments, as they are currently performed, date only to the early 1970s. Economic evaluation is supposed to produce information that might lead to better economic decisions, meaning that scarce resources in health care are allocated in the most efficient way. Although economic evaluation is designed to support decision making, the actual influence of economic evaluation in policy decisions leaves much to be desired. One of the reasons for this suboptimal use of information from economic evaluations is the use of a variety of methodologies in different studies, which hampers comparability between studies. Therefore, a good deal of effort has been put into the development of standardised methods for economic evaluations. At present, textbooks[1] and consensus books[2] exist, and numerous country-specific (pharmacoeconomic) guidelines provide detailed recommendations on how best to perform an economic evaluation. Although there is consensus on major issues related to economic evaluations, recent debates in the literature have shown that disagreements still persist on many other issues (for example, on the measurement of production loss, the use of utility assessments and/or willingness to pay).

Guidelines can serve many purposes.[3] First, guidelines can be linked to a formal requirement to provide economic data before a new technology is accepted. The development and application of pharmacoeconomic guidelines is an important example in this category. Second, guidelines can set methodological standards that researchers should meet in making economic evaluations. Finally, guidelines could contain ethical standards for the practice of economic evaluation (good economic practice analogous to good clinical practice).

A further development is the intensified use of systematic reviews and meta-analyses to summarise knowledge and provide "state-of-the-art" evidence in a certain area.[4] A systematic review produces an overview of studies (usually selected from the published literature) on a specific topic and synthesising summaries and conclusions on therapeutic effectiveness, diagnostic information, or aetiological and prognostic factors. Systematic reviews usually contain qualitative information, accounting for the methodological quality of the included studies. Meta-analysis is the quantitative method of combining the results of studies on a specific topic (also called statistical pooling). The results of the individual studies are statistically combined to provide an overall measure or pooled estimate of the (cost-)effectiveness of a health care intervention.

Originally, the methodology of performing systematic reviews comes from the field of psychology. Health care methodologists, like biostatisticians and epidemiologists, took the initiative in developing and adapting the methods of systematic reviews in the field of health care. They developed statistical methods for pooling data from different research settings. They also developed a methodology to assess the quality of the studies performed, using criteria for quality.[5,6] In reviewing the existing literature, one finds in many cases studies that show more or less conflicting results. The consequent challenge is to consider and take into account the validity of the individual studies, and come to a final conclusion on the overall outcome.

This process of meta-analysis and systematic review of RCTs on effectiveness, including assessment of the quality of the individual studies, has become a well-developed area in the field of clinical studies over the past ten years. Criteria for quality encompass both internal validity (design, conduct and analysis) and external validity (generalisability). Furthermore, the quality of reporting is important as the reviews are usually based on published studies. Moher and colleagues showed that poor reporting is associated with overestimation of treatment effects.[5,6]

A large number of instruments exist to assess the methodological quality of effect studies.[5,6] Best known are the criteria list developed by Thomas Chalmers[7], the Jadad list[8] and the Delphi list by Verhagen.[9] One study compared 25 different instruments for assessing the quality of RCTs by applying them to one review.[10] The results differed substantially, indicating that the content of the criteria list influences the outcome and is therefore of utmost importance.

Although a large number of systematic reviews of economic evaluations have been performed to date, the methodology in this field is less well developed. One of the reasons is that economic evaluation studies may be even more diverse than effectiveness studies. A number of guidelines for assessing the quality of economic evaluations in systematic reviews have been developed and published. One of these lists was developed by members of the ☑ CHEC project and was used in several systematic reviews of economic evaluations.[11–14] Common problems encountered in these systematic reviews arose from the low number of available studies, the low quality of the data and the poor methodology used within these studies. Regarding the quantity, it was striking that, in general, despite the increased interest in economic evaluation, rather few full economic evaluation studies have been undertaken. In addition, only a limited number of these studies could be classified as cost-utility studies, using quality-adjusted life years (QALYs) as the outcome measure. As to cost calculations, although it is widely recommended, especially from a societal perspective, to include a wide range of costs, only a few studies included all relevant costs. Furthermore, the methods used for cost measurement and cost valuation were often unclear. Almost all studies were "piggybacked", as appendices to the medical outcome study, with the consequence that a separate power analysis regarding economic outcome parameters was not performed in any of the studies. Based on these observations, the reviews concluded that the quality of the studies included was very low.

The lack of a generally accepted methodology for reviewing the economic literature can be considered one of the primary reasons why economic evaluations do not have much influence on policy making. Consequently the ☑ CHEC project aims to enhance the informativeness of reviews of economic evaluations by developing a criteria list which can be used for a solid systematic review regarding such studies. Such a list could be combined with one of the existing criteria lists for assessing the quality of the clinical part of the studies (usually and preferably the randomised controlled trial), in order to assess the overall methodological quality of the clinical study.

Guidelines, checklists and criteria lists

Guidelines give instructions on how to adequately perform or report a study. A researcher performing a cost-effectiveness analysis (CEA) may use guidelines in designing and conducting a study. A checklist is used after the study has been performed and after the results have been published to see if the study met specific guidelines. Of course, there will be a large overlap between guidelines and checklists for the same type of studies.

Criteria lists are used in systematic reviews to consider the methodological quality of the studies included. The criteria usually relate to the internal validity of the studies, but in some criteria lists external validity items are also included. Obviously, different criteria are relevant to different types of studies and different criteria lists should be used for the methodological quality assessment of, for example, randomised trials, or of economic or observational studies. Again, there may be some overlap between criteria lists and guidelines or checklists in a specific research field, but criteria lists are usually more compact and serve a different purpose. That is, the methodological quality assessed by a criteria list should indicate how high or low the chance is that the results of the study are inaccurate or misleading.

Development of a criteria list for the assessment of the methodological quality of economic evaluations in systematic reviews

General design

The aim of the ☑ CHEC project is to develop a criteria list to be used in systematic reviews of economic evaluation studies, by identifying a minimum set of methodological items that reflect the methodological quality of individual economic evaluation studies. The ultimate goal is to produce a systematic, uniform and sound approach to systematic reviews of economic evaluations, so that readers of systematic reviews have the opportunity to judge the quality of the economic evaluation studies included, and have some insight into the validity and reliability of the outcomes. The ☑ CHEC project will focus on the methodological quality of economic evaluations (for example, costs and effects), because other checklists already focus on the methodological quality of more general aspects of clinical effectiveness studies (see Appendix 8.1).

The criteria list has been developed using the Delphi method. This is a consensus method, making use of experts who give written opinions and arguments on a specific problem. These arguments are exchanged among the members of the Delphi panel and this process is repeated until consensus is reached or no new information comes up.[15,16]

Choice of experts

A large number of international experts participated in the Delphi panel. First a Task Force Group was formed consisting of seven internationally acknowledged and prominent experts in the field of economic evaluation. This Task Force Group assisted the project team (authors of this chapter) with the composition of the final Delphi panel. Participants for the Delphi panel were selected if they were authors of guidelines or checklists or if they had special expertise in economic evaluation studies. The project team made a first selection, keeping a balance between various countries and research groups. The inclusion of experts from different research settings all over the world was an explicit goal. This was considered essential for reaching broad acceptance and support for the final criteria list. This preliminary list of experts was evaluated by the Task Force Group, which could suggest eliminating or accepting proposed experts or suggest new candidates for the Delphi panel. This procedure resulted in a final list of 17 persons who were invited to the Delphi panel (See Appendix 8.2). The members of the Task Force Group also participated in the Delphi panel, leading to a final complete panel of 24 members.

Selection of items

Items were selected from existing guidelines, checklists and criteria lists regarding cost-effectiveness analysis. Several strategies were combined to identify the relevant literature in the field of economic evaluation. First, a MEDLINE search was performed for the period 1990 to 2000 using MeSH headings "cost and cost analysis", "meta-analysis" or "review literature". Additionally, Psychlit and Econlit were screened for the same period using keywords "review" or "meta-analysis" and "economic" or "cost*" in titles. Additional articles were identified by searching the Cochrane Library (2000, Issue 3) and the NHS EED database using the terms "cost*" or "economic*". Finally, handbooks on economic evaluation studies were monitored and a request to submit additional guidelines was presented to the Healthecon Discussion List.

Analysis of existing guidelines

A total of 25 guidelines were initially identified through the procedure described above (see Appendix 8.3). A closer look revealed that several guidelines were the same and others were inadequate for our goal. Thus, 15 different guidelines (see Table 8.1) were finally included, which were used for the first item selection.

There was still a wide variety among these 15 guidelines. Some of the guidelines aimed at providing information to researchers, others at providing information to journal referees or to authors who intend to submit their study for publication in journals. Some guidelines restricted themselves to about 10 items, using very broadly defined items, whereas other guidelines produced lists of up to 50 detailed items. In Table 8.1 these guidelines are described in more detail. A distinction was made between: (1) guidelines for economic evaluations and (2) guidelines for performing systematic reviews or assessment of published studies.

Six guidelines were developed for economic evaluations and nine for systematic reviews. In general, little attention has been paid to the following aspects: description of target population, follow up period and the independent position of investigators. The first two aspects could be considered methodological aspects. The independence of the investigator seems to be recognised as a relevant factor in some of the more recent guidelines. Aspects covered by many guidelines are standard economic evaluation core issues like: choice of alternatives, perspective, identification measurement and valuation of costs and benefits, discounting, handling of uncertainties and application of incremental analysis.

Designing the Delphi survey

Preparing the questionnaire for the first Delphi round

The initial item pool was constructed using the items of the 15 guidelines (see Table 8.1), so that there was a total of 218 items. Unavoidably, there were many duplicate items and this first item pool was somewhat redundant. The item pool was restructured by: (1) development of a classification scheme and (2) reduction of the item pool.

Table 8.1 Analysis of 15 existing guidelines.

	Category	Guidelines for economic evaluation						Guidelines for systematic reviews								
		Adams	Clemens	Detsky	Eisenberg	Gerard	Gold	Bradley Gibson Sacristán	MUHSC Drummond 1996 Drummond 1997	Drummond 1997	Drummond 1993	Evers	Haycox	Lee	Sanchez 1995 Sanchez 1999	Udvarhelyi
1	Description of the target population		×				×	×	×		×					
2	Choice of alternatives	×	×	×	×		×	×	×	×	×		×	×	×	
3	Economic study question		×	×		×		×	×		×	×		×	×	
4	Economic study design	×		×	×		×	×	×		×	×			×	
5	Follow up period		×		×		×	×			×					
6	Perspective	×	×	×	×	×	×	×	×			×			×	×
7	Economic identification	×	×	×	×				×		×	×		×	×	×
8	Economic measurement	×		×	×	×		×	×	×	×	×		×	×	
9	Economic valuation	×		×	×	×			×	×	×	×		×	×	
10	Outcome identification	×	×	×			×		×		×	×		×	×	×
11	Outcome measurement	×		×	×	×	×	×	×	×	×	×		×		
12	Outcome valuation			×		×			×	×	×	×		×	×	
13	Adjustment for time variation	×	×		×	×	×	×	×		×	×		×	×	×
14	Sensitivity and uncertainties	×	×	×	×	×	×	×	×	×	×	×		×	×	×
15	Presentation of results			×		×	×	×	×		×				×	×
16	Generalisability of results		×			×	×		×	×	×		×		×	
17	Incremental analysis	×	×	×	×		×	×	×	×	×	×		×	×	×
18	Independence of investigators			×											×	
19	Ethics and distribution of effects	×		×	×		×	×	×							

For references see Appendix 8.3

Development of a classification scheme

To facilitate analysis of the item pool, a classification scheme was developed for the individual items. This classification was a necessary step in order to reduce the number of items in a scientifically justified way, without any loss of information. Three members of the team (SE, MG and AA) developed a classification scheme in a rather open consensus procedure. Starting with broad categories (for example, "costs" and "benefits"), categories were added if new items could not be classified into one of the categories that were used at that moment. If there were many items in one category and subdivision was considered necessary, subcategories were created. For example, the category "costs" was subdivided into the classes "identification of costs", "measurement of costs" and "valuation of costs". Finally, a classification scheme with 19 categories was developed, in which almost all items of the original pool could be classified (see Table 8.1).

However, some items were difficult to classify. When there was no consensus among the three investigators about classification, these items were provisionally put into a separate category labelled "unclear".

Reduction of the item pool

Reduction of items should be performed in a transparent and reproducible way. A two-step method was applied to complete this reduction:

1 Items were first classified into several subcategories. For example, for the subcategory "measuring costs": in some guidelines the item was phrased "How are costs measured?", whereas in other guidelines the question was slightly differently phrased as "Are costs measured appropriately?", and in other guidelines even more specifically "Are costs measured suitably for the perspective?". Careful analysis of the items in the subcategories led to further subdivision. The final items for the first Delphi round were presented using this more refined classification.
2 After classifying the items according to this more detailed system, it became possible to compare more or less similar items directly with each other, which facilitated further reduction of the item pool without any loss of information.

The following strategy was used for item reduction:

1 No items on general methodology (covered by criteria lists of clinical trials).
2 (Almost) identical formulations skipped.
3 More general wording preferred above specific wording.
4 No double questions are allowed.

5 No use of the word "should".
6 "Closed" items are better than "open" items.
7 No unclear, imprecise items.
8 Item must be clear and understandable, without original context.
9 Items must be clear, without examples.
10 Short wording is preferred over extensive wording.
11 Objective items are preferred over subjective items.
12 Present time is preferred over past time in wording.

After applying the above rules to the initial item pool, the number of items reduced from 218 to 128. This set of 128 items was used in the first Delphi round.

Phrasing of answering categories

Of course, the phrasing of the answering categories is related to the way the original questions were phrased. In the original guidelines, all kinds of answering categories were found, and these categories sometimes varied even within one guideline. Although the majority of questions were formulated in a more closed or objective way – asking for dichotomous answers (Yes/No), asking for hard evidence or objective information (for example: "Are costs discounted?") – in many other cases the questions were phrased in a more open or subjective way (for example: "Are costs discounted appropriately?"), with questions asking for interpretations from a broader perspective (for example: "Are costs measured appropriately for the research question?"). Sometimes rather limited enumeration of answering categories was provided; for example, in determining the perspective of the analysis (society, the health care sector, insurers, institutions, clients, other). In other cases, categorical answering categories were used; for example, the item concerning whether costs were measured appropriately could consist of four answering categories: all (all costs are measured appropriately), most, some and none.

In the first Delphi round, we asked the panel only if they considered the items to be relevant as appropriate elements of the criteria list, but did not ask about the specific answering categories.

Design of the first Delphi round

The questionnaire of the first Delphi round was returned by 23 of the 24 experts who were selected for the Delphi panel. The questionnaire consisted of 128 items spread over 19 categories. First, the expert was asked to state for each category whether it should be included in a criteria list of a minimum set of items. Then, the expert was asked to give his or her opinion about the items in each of the categories that they wanted on the list, regarding whether these items should be on the list. Furthermore, it was possible for the expert to give an alternative formulation for an item.

Table 8.2 Responses of the first Delphi round.

Categories		Agreement on inclusion of category (%)	Number of items within each category	Agreement on inclusion of individual items (%)
1	Description of the target population	100	2	55–77
2	Choice of alternatives	100	7	17–91
3	Economic study question	91	2	39–87
4	Economic study design	91	3	26–70
5	Follow up period	100	2	61–83
6	Perspective	100	3	43–78
7	Resource use/input identification	100	11	22–78
8	Resource use/input measurement	96	19	9–57
9	Resource use/input valuation	96	10	9–57
10	Outcome identification	100	10	30–78
11	Outcome measurement	96	8	26–65
12	Outcome valuation	96	4	35–65
13	Discounting/adjustment for time differences	100	7	43–70
14	Sensitivity and uncertainties	100	8	22–78
15	Presentation of results	100	10	30–96
16	Generalisability of results	91	5	17–87
17	Incremental analysis	87	8	13–70
18	Independence of investigators	91	1	83
19	Ethics and distributional effects	83	3	26–61

Results of the Delphi round

The results of the first Delphi round showed that the differences for each category were minimal (see Table 8.2). However, the items did show some obvious differences (see Table 8.2). The experts influenced the analysis, since they judged the items not only in a quantitative way, but also in a qualitative way. The alternative formulations for the items that the experts suggested presented some problems, as a simple quantitative analysis (by using a cut-off point of the percentage of responses) was no longer sufficient. Each separate category of the questionnaire was analysed, to evaluate the percentage as well as the alternative formulations that were suggested by the experts.

In general, there is a high agreement on the categories to be included in the final version of the ☑ CHEC list. This can be concluded from the second column of Table 8.2. For example, all of the experts have the opinion that "Description of the target population" (first category) should be represented in the final criteria list. There is less agreement with regard to item 17, "Incremental analysis" (87%) and 19 "Ethics and distributional effects" (83%).

However, if one looks at the range of the responses on the separate items within each category, there is much less consensus among the experts. This can be seen from the third and fourth columns. For example, category 1 contains two items: in the fourth column there is a range from 55 to77%, which means that 55% of the experts agree on the one item and 77% agree on the other item. In the second Delphi round the focus will be on these differences in order to construct the final criteria list. This is even more complicated because there are also additional suggestions given by some experts in the first round which are not reported on here.

Conclusion and discussions

By creating a criteria list consisting of a minimum set of items, the ☑ CHEC project makes it possible for future systematic reviews of economic evaluations to become more transparent, informative and comparable. Consequently, these systematic reviews might be used more easily by researchers and policy makers. However, the project has some limitations, as follows.

The ☑ CHEC criteria list does not include more general design characteristics of clinical studies, because criteria lists for these aspects have already been published in the international literature. In the future, the ☑ CHEC criteria list might be combined with a criteria list concerning effect studies.[5,7,9]

The possible combination of the ☑ CHEC list with another list raises an additional point. The other lists clearly are only applicable in randomised or non-randomised controlled trials (RCTs and CCTs respectively). Economic evaluations very often do make use of other designs. Use of the ☑ CHEC list in combination with another existing list is therefore limited to full economic evaluations alongside RCTs or CCTs. The RCT design is considered to be the gold standard within the field of evidence-based medicine, but it is widely recognised that in many situations this design cannot be used. Economic evaluations are also based on modelling studies, in which a wide variety of data gathering techniques and data processing models are used. There is still a need to develop an additional checklist for assessing the quality of economic evaluations based on modelling studies or other designs.

Guidelines have been criticised because of their potential rigidity, which might prohibit further development of methodology. This criticism is only valid if guidelines are used injudiciously. To prevent the criteria list from being methodologically rigid, it should be emphasised that this list is a minimum set, with the aim of stimulating researchers to add additional items appropriate for the specific subject under study.

Many of the experts that we asked to participate in the Delphi panel gave their consent. One refused because he was concerned that the development of a criteria list would lead to disregard of low quality studies that might nevertheless contain useful information in some sense, and that sometimes it might be better to base decisions on less optimal information than on no information at all. In this context, it is important to emphasise that the aim of our criteria list is to describe the characteristics of all studies retrieved and not to throw studies away or ignore information. Including quality assessment when using this criteria list may help decision makers (and others) to recognise the validity of the studies and the usefulness of the information.

In order eventually to reach broad acceptance among the scientific community a Delphi panel of widely acknowledged persons was composed. In this chapter the first step of the procedure has been reported; the second Delphi round has yet to be undertaken and it is only after the second step that the final list of criteria will be produced. Additionally, in order to stimulate dissemination of the criteria list a validation procedure of the final list will be undertaken.

Finally, there are many examples of poor reporting in economic evaluation studies. It is often difficult to conclude what actually happened in the study and this affects the methodological quality assessment. A solution could be to contact the authors of the original paper, asking them for a more detailed description of the study design. An alternative would be to require the production of a standard technical report for every economic evaluation study. This technical report should be available for everyone, on the Internet if possible. Such a technical report, describing the economic design of the study, could then be used in the systematic review. The criteria list has the potential to influence the quality of both the performance and the reporting of economic evaluation studies.

Hopefully the ☑ CHEC project will lead to a generally acceptable criteria list for the methodological quality assessment of economic evaluations in systematic reviews. The adoption of such a core set of items by researchers could lead to increased comparability of the results of systematic reviews of economic evaluation studies in the near future.

Appendices

Appendix 8.1: Methodological criteria list for systematic reviews[9]

1 Was a method of randomisation performed?
2 Was the treatment allocation concealed?
3 Were the groups similar at baseline regarding most important prognostic factors?
4 Were the eligibility criteria specified?
5 Was the outcome assessor blinded?
6 Was the care provider blinded?
7 Was the patient blinded?
8 Were point estimates and measures of variability presented for the primary outcome measures?
9 Did the analysis include an intention-to-treat analysis?

Answering categories: Yes/No/Don't know

Appendix 8.2: Members of the Task Force Group and the Delphi panel of the ☑ CHEC project

Prof MJ Buxton	Brunel University (UK)	Task Force
Mr D Coyle	Ottawa Civic Hospital (Canada)	Task Force
Prof MF Drummond	University of York (UK)	Task Force
Dr AE Elixhauser	Center for Organization and Delivery Studies (US)	Task Force
Prof E Jonsson	Swedish Council on Health Technology Assessment	Task Force
Prof M Mugford	University of East Anglia and Cochrane Health Economics Methods Group (UK)	Task Force
Prof FFH Rutten	Erasmus University (Netherlands)	Delphi Panel
Prof DH Banta	TNO (Netherlands)	Delphi Panel
Prof C Donaldson	University of Calgary (Canada)	Delphi Panel
Prof B Jönsson	Stockholm School of Economics (Sweden)	Delphi Panel
Prof K Kesteloot	KU Leuven (Belgium)	Delphi Panel
Dr BR Luce	MEDTAP International Inc. (US)	Delphi Panel
Dr G Lyman	The Cancer Center (US)	Delphi Panel
Dr D Menon	Institute of Health Economics (Canada)	Delphi Panel
Dr E Nord	National Institute of Public Health (Norway)	Delphi Panel
Prof B O'Brien	St. Joseph's Hospital, McMaster University, Hamilton (Canada)	Delphi Panel
Prof J Rovira	Soikos SL (Spain)	Delphi Panel
Prof LB Russell	Rutgers University (US)	Delphi Panel
Dr G Simon	Group Health Cooperative, Washington (US)	Delphi Panel
Prof JE Sisk	Mount Sinai School of Medicine, New York City (US)	Delphi Panel
Dr R Taylor	National Institute for Clinical Excellence (UK)	Delphi Panel
Prof GW Torrance	McMaster University (Canada)	Delphi Panel
Mr A Towse	Office of Health Economics (UK)	Delphi Panel
Mr L Vale	University of Aberdeen, Scotland (UK)	Delphi Panel

Appendix 8.3: List of guidelines examined

*Adams ME, McCall NT, Gray DT, Orza MJ, Chalmers TC. Economic analysis in randomized control trials. *Med Care* 1992;**30**:231–43.

Blackmore CC, Magid DJ. Methodologic evaluation of the radiology cost-effectiveness literature (see comments). *Radiology* 1997;**203**:87–91.

*Bradley CA, Iskedjian M, Lanctôt KL, Mittman N, Simone C, St Pierre E. Quality assessment of economic evaluations in selected pharmacy, medical, and health economic journals. *Ann Pharmacother* 1995;**29**:681–9.

Buxton MA. *The Canadian experience: step change or gradual evolution?* London: Office of Health Economics, 1997.

*Clemens K, Townsend R, Luscombe F, Mauskopf J, Osterhaus J, Bobula J. Methodological and conduct principles for pharmacoeconomic research. *Pharmacoeconomics* 1995; **8**:169–74.

*Department of Clinical Epidemiology and Biostatistics MUHSC. How to read clinical journals: VII. To understand an economic evaluation (part B). *Can Med Assoc J* 1984; **130**:1542–9.

*Detsky AS. Guidelines for economic analysis of pharmaceutical products. A draft document for Ontario and Canada. *Pharmacoeconomics* 1993;**3**:354–61.

*Drummond M. User's guides to the medical literature: XIII. How to use an article on economic analysis of clinical practice. *JAMA* 1997;**277**:552–6.

*Drummond M, Brandt A, Luce B, Rovira J. Standardizing methodologies for economic evaluation in health care. *Int J Technol Assess Health Care* 1993;**9**:26–36.

*Drummond MF, Jefferson TO. Guidelines for authors and peer reviewers of economic submissions to the *BMJ*. The BMJ Economic Evaluation Working Party. *BMJ* 1996; **313**:275–83.

*Drummond MF, O'Brien BJ, Stoddart GL, Torrance GW. *Methods for the economic evaluation of health care programmes*, 2nd edn. Oxford: Oxford University Press, 1997.

*Eisenberg JM. Clinical economics. A guide to economic analysis of clinical practices. *JAMA* 1989;**262**:2879–86.

*Evers SMAA, Wijk AS, Ament AJHA. Economic evaluations of mental health care interventions. A review. Internal report, University of Maastricht, Department of Health Economics, 1994, p 39.

Ganiats TG, Wong AF. Evaluation of cost-effectiveness research. A survey of recent publications. *Family Med* 1991;**23**:457–61.

*Gerard K. Cost-utility in practice: a policy maker's guide to the state of the art. *Health Policy* 1992;**21**:249–79.

*Gibson GA. Use of the guidelines to evaluate and interpret pharmacoeconomic literature. Pharmacoeconomics and outcomes. Internal report, Kansas City, American College of Clinical Pharmacy, 1996, pp 325–64.

*Gold MR, Russell LB, Siegel JE, Weinstein MC. *Cost-effectiveness in health and medicine.* Oxford: Oxford University Press, 1996.

*Haycox A, Drummond M, Walley T. Pharmacoeconomics: integrating economic evaluation into clinical trials. *Br J Clin Pharmacol* 1997;**43**:559–62.

*Lee JT, Sanchez LA. Interpretation of "cost-effective" and soundness of economic evaluations in the pharmacy literature. *Am J Hosp Pharmacol* 1991;**48**:2622–7.

Mason J, Drummond M. Reporting guidelines for economic studies. *Health Econ* 1995;**4**:85–94.

*Sacristán JA, Soto J, Galende I. Evaluation of pharmacoeconomic studies: utilization of a checklist. *Ann Pharmacother* 1993;**27**:1126–33.

*Sanchez LA. Evaluating the quality of published pharmacoeconomic evaluations. *Hosp Pharm* 1995;**30**:146–8.

*Sanchez LA. Applied pharmacoeconomics: evaluation and use of pharmacoeconomic data from the literature. *Am J Health-system Pharm* 1999;**56**:1630–8.

Task Force on Principles for Economic Analysis of Health Care Technology. Economic analysis of health care technology. A report on principles. *Ann Intern Med* 1995;**123**:61–70.

*Udvarhelyi S, Colditz GA, Rai A, Epstein AM. Cost-effectiveness and cost-benefit analysis in the medical literature. *Ann Intern Med* 1992;**116**:238–44.

*Denotes items producing the final 15 different guidelines selected for the first Delphi round.

References

References for the guidelines examined are given in Appendix 8.2.

1 Drummond MF, O'Brien B, Stoddart GL, Torrance GW. *Methods for the economic evaluation of health care programmes*. Oxford: Oxford University Press, 1997.
2 Gold M, Siegel JE, Russell LB, Weinstein MC. *Cost-effectiveness in health and medicine*. Oxford: Oxford University Press, 1996.
3 Drummond MF. Guidelines for pharmacoeconomic studies: the ways forward. *Pharmacoeconomics* 1994;**6**:493–7.
4 Mulrow CD, Langhorne P, Grimshaw J. Integrating heterogeneous pieces of evidence in systematic reviews. *Ann Intern Med* 1997;**127**:989–95.
5 Moher D, Jadad A, Tugwell P. Assessing the quality of randomized controlled trials. Current issues and future directions. *Int J Technol Assess Health Care* 1996;**12**:195–208.
6 Moher D, Pham BA, Jones A. Does quality of reports of randomised trials affect estimates of intervention efficacy reported in meta-analyses? *Lancet* 1998;**352**:609–13.
7 Chalmers TC, Smith H, Jr, Blackburn B, Silverman B, Schroeder B, Reitman D *et al.* A method for assessing the quality of a randomized control trial. *Control Clin Trials* 1981;**2**:231–49.
8 Jadad A, Moore R, Carroll D, Jenkinson C, Reynolds J, McQuay H. Assessing the quality of reports of randomized clinical trials: is blinding necessary? *Control Clin Trials* 1996;**17**:1–12.
9 Verhagen A, de Vet H, de Bie R, Kessels A, Boers M, Bouter L *et al.* The Delphi list: a criteria list for quality assessment of randomized clinical trials for conducting systematic reviews developed by Delphi consensus. *J Clin Epidemiol* 1998;**51**:1235–41.
10 Juni P, Witschi A, Bloch R, Egger M. The hazards of scoring the quality of clinical trials for meta-analysis. *JAMA* 1999;**11**:1054–60.
11 Evers SM, Van Wijk AS, Ament AJ. Economic evaluation of mental health care interventions. A review. *Health Econ* 1997;**6**:161–77.
12 Evers SM, Ament AJ, Blaauw G. Economic evaluation of patients with cerebrovascular diseases: a review. *Stroke* 2000;**31**:1046–53.
13 Goossens M, Evers SM. Economic assessment of back pain interventions. *J Occup Rehab* 1997;**7**:15–32.
14 Goossens M, Evers SM. Cost-effectiveness of treatment of neck and low back pain. In: Nachemson A, Jonsson E, eds. *Neck and back pain. The scientific evidence of causes, diagnosis and treatment.* Stockholm/Philadelphia: SBU/Lippincott, 2000.
15 Delbecq AL, Van de Ven AH, Gustafson DH, Foreman S. *Group techniques for program planning: a guide to nominal group technique and Delphi processes*. Glenview: 1975.
16 Whitman N. The Delphi technique as an alternative for committee meetings. *J Nurs Educ* 1990;**29**:377–9.

9: Evaluating economic interventions: a role for non-randomised designs?

IVAR SØNBØ KRISTIANSEN, TOBY GOSDEN

Introduction

Systematic reviews are proposed as an efficient means of integrating valid information to facilitate rational decision making.[1] While systematic reviews traditionally have been used to analyse choice of medical treatments, they can be used to obtain the "best" available evidence to answer health policy questions about economic interventions such as doctor payment systems.[2,3] The area of doctor payment systems has been well researched.[4,5] However, despite this abundance there still remains much uncertainty surrounding the effects of different payments systems because the studies vary so much with respect to context, type of incentives, study design and data quality.

Such payment systems will be used as a case study in this chapter, where the authors' experience of carrying out two systematic reviews for the Effective Practice and Organisation of Care (EPOC) review group of the Cochrane Collaboration is described.[6] The impact of different payment systems on doctor behaviour is examined. The main results of the reviews are reported, followed by discussions of how the utility of the findings to policy makers is limited by the nature of the evidence base.

A case study of reviews on the impact of payment methods on primary care physician behaviour

Two reviews were conducted[7,8] of studies evaluating the impact of different methods of payment on primary care physician (PCP) behaviour.

One review covered the three most prevalent payment systems – capitation, salary and fee-for-service (FFS) – and another covered target payments, which is a relatively new remuneration system and is of policy interest in both the USA and UK. The reviews sought to determine whether doctors respond to the financial incentives generated by these different types of payment systems.

These different methods are hypothesised to provide very different incentives. Under capitation, the doctor receives income in the form of a payment for each registered patient. This payment may cover some or all services a patient may receive. Salaried doctors receive a lump sum salary, which is independent of the number of services they provide, number of patients registered with them or hours they work. FFS pays doctors a fee for each item or unit of care they provide, for example, immunisations, types of consultations and prescriptions. Target payment is a form of FFS where doctors are remunerated if, and only if, they reach a certain target *level* of service (such as numbers of patients covered by an immunisation programme).

A narrow focus was chosen for both of the reviews because of the size and nature of the evidence base on payment systems. The focus was on PCPs, the interest being in obtaining evidence of the effect of payment systems on objective measures of the following: professional satisfaction with their working environment; the cost, quantity, type and pattern of care; equity of care; and clinical outcomes of care. Copies were obtained of the papers of 332 references thought to be relevant from a total of 5499 references found using the search strategy,[9] and two reviewers assessed whether each article met the inclusion criteria in the usual way.

Only those study designs that were acceptable according to the EPOC criteria were included,[10] and, thus, three randomised controlled trials (RCTs), two controlled before and after studies and one interrupted time series (ITS) were found. The findings of each study could not be statistically pooled because of the heterogeneity in outcomes measured and settings. Furthermore, because of the diverse nature of the interventions themselves it was important to describe the specific contexts of each study, and to review the results in the light of the objectives of the change in payment system and the expectations of the authors.

Appendices 9.1 and 9.2 highlight the heterogeneous nature of the studies included in the reviews. The PCPs involved in all the evaluations except the Krasnik and Ritchie studies were volunteers. The studies varied in sample size, with the smallest number of PCPs being 18 in the Hickson study and the largest being 426 in the Krasnik study. Sample size calculations were not reported in any of the studies but even in the smallest there were statistically significant findings. Of the three trials, two met one out of the six methodological criteria (see Gosden *et al*[8]), whilst the remaining study met four. In two of the three trials, there were unit of analysis errors, in that randomisation was done at one level (for example, the practice) whilst analysis was conducted at a less aggregate level (for example, the doctor). These errors make confidence intervals appear smaller than they actually are, leading to erroneous conclusions. The Hutchison study met all six criteria for controlled before and after designs, whereas the Krasnik study met only two. The only ITS study met all the quality criteria except having the sufficient number (12) of observations before and after the intervention to enable reliable statistical inference; there were 12 before but only 6 after. As the Appendices show, inadequate reporting of study details rather than low methodological quality was the main reason why some of the studies did not meet all the criteria. In addition, few studies reported information on important confounding factors such as PCP and patient characteristics.

Capitation versus FFS

The trial carried out in New York, USA by Davidson *et al* compared paediatricians paid by capitation with two groups paid by FFS, with one group of FFS physicians (intervention group 2) having higher levels of fees than the control FFS group.[11,12] The logic behind these interventions was that low fees and unstable client eligibility discouraged FFS doctors from providing care to patients. Consequently patients were receiving care directly from more expensive hospital providers. The study sought to determine whether prepayment (capitation) or higher fees would contain costs whilst maintaining access to care. Although not explicitly stated by the authors, increasing fees yield cost savings presumably by encouraging a switch from expensive hospital providers to primary care. However, the capitation and FFS group fees were set at a level designed to provide the same income to PCPs with the same number of patients and/or service provision. Therefore, it seemed to us that the authors were comparing the effect of both the type of payment as well as the level of income in the study.

These "hypotheses" were broadly in line with expectations in that where services are financed by capitation payments this would encourage physicians to use smaller quantities of services than if these services were linked to fees.[13] Physicians paid by capitation who are at risk for all the services they recommend, as was the case in this trial, would be expected to substitute the most expensive (hospital) services with the least (primary care).[14] Additionally, higher fees would be expected to increase the profitability of providing care thus encouraging PCPs to treat patients.[15,16]

Logistic regression was used to control for higher baseline levels of service utilisation and demographic differences in the patient populations. The authors estimated two regression models: one explaining utilisation during the project, and one explaining the change in utilisation from the before intervention period to during the project. If the coefficients for the intervention payment variables were statistically significant in both models the authors argued this was strong evidence of an effect. Using this argument there was strong evidence that capitation payment was associated with fewer non-PCP visits but only weak evidence that more PCP visits had taken place and that there were fewer emergency room visits and hospitalisations compared with the control FFS group. The evidence that the higher fee intervention was associated with more PCP visits was strong but there was no evidence that the number of hospitalisations and non-PCP visits fell, although there was weak evidence that there were fewer visits to the emergency clinic. This finding may have been because the physicians in the higher fee intervention group had no financial incentive or disincentive to alter the provision of these services.

The authors used regression to estimate the estimated effects of the two interventions on changes in expenditure on the different types of visits. As would be expected from the more robust findings above, capitation resulted in lower expenditure on non-PCP visits; however, both capitation and higher fees increased expenditure on PCP services compared with the control FFS group. Expenditure on hospital and emergency services was unaffected by the two payment interventions, despite weak evidence that capitation affected the *number* of hospitalisations.

A study carried out in Denmark evaluated the introduction of fees in the existing capitation payment system of GPs in Copenhagen City.[17–19] Fees were introduced principally to compensate GPs in Copenhagen for decreasing levels of income and rising workload, compared with GPs outside Copenhagen already being paid by capitation and FFS. Krasnik *et al* hypothesised that GPs seek to achieve a target level of income[20] rather than to maximise income.[21] It was assumed that GPs in Copenhagen City had income levels below their target levels before the introduction of fees and that afterwards GPs would increase their activity, especially where they had most discretion, in order to try to meet this target. Fees for providing primary care services only would have the opposite effect to capitation payment for primary care;[22,23] therefore, the authors expected GPs to substitute their own time for hospital care and referrals to specialists and hospitals to fall. The study authors also expected that GPs would "overshoot" their target initially and then adjust activity levels downwards, perhaps directing their effort towards the most profitable services,[16] until they reached their target.

Krasnik *et al* controlled for the number of persons enlisted and differences in the level of activity of the doctors in their analysis. The results are largely consistent with the expectations of the authors. The activity levels of four out of the five services remunerated by the new fees increased in the first year after the change to levels higher than those generated by GPs outside Copenhagen. The fall in the renewal of prescriptions was thought to have been due to the lower profitability of this service compared with others. As predicted, referral rates fell after the change and were lower than amongst non-city GPs. Two out of the five services linked to fees initially rose and then fell 18 months after the payment change, whereas diagnostic and curative services continued to rise to levels substantially above those provided by GPs outside the city.

A confounding factor that could not be controlled for in the analysis was the concurrent increase in contracted hours worked by Copenhagen GPs. However, the authors argue that the increase in activity levels was attributable to a greater number of services being provided per patient rather than an increase in the number of patients. Also, the authors suggested that the study might have underestimated the effects of the fees as the GPs involved in the study were expected to be less sensitive to financial incentives compared with non-participating GPs.

Mixed capitation versus FFS

Health Service Organisations (HSOs) in Ontario, Canada remunerate PCPs by capitation. A policy objective of the HSO programme was to reduce hospital utilisation by encouraging more preventive care and the substitution of primary care for hospital services. The Ambulatory Care Incentive Plan (ACIP) was introduced to provide a financial reward to those HSOs for every day that hospital utilisation (hospital days per 1000 patients adjusted for age and sex) was below the average for the municipality, district or region. This payment provides a direct financial incentive to constrain hospitalisation, and capitation, if it covers expenditure on hospital use, also provides a cost-containment incentive.[14] Hutchison *et al* aimed to test whether PCPs switching from FFS payment (pre-HSO) to capitation and ACIP payments had lower rates of hospitalisation.[24] They also tested whether HSO PCPs changed their behaviour in anticipation of the change from FFS to capitation/ACIP.

The authors tracked HSO PCPs who had previously worked in FFS practice (non-HSO) and compared hospitalisation rates before and after the physician joined the HSO and with hospital use amongst physicians who remained in FFS practice. The authors matched HSO and FFS PCPs by a number of personal, job and practice/area characteristics (see Appendices). The study authors found that hospitalisation rates did not change amongst PCPs either before or after joining the HSO. The study authors suggested that the results were partially due to limited hospital bed availability and the lack of influence PCPs had over hospital admission and discharge decisions, which were increasingly being made by hospital specialists.

An additional consideration was that the HSO programme may have attracted PCPs with particular preferences or characteristics that were related to their clinical behaviour (that is, selection bias), which the matching and analysis was unable to control for. For example, low referring PCPs would benefit financially from the programme and so these would be more likely to join. However, the authors suggest that this would have been more likely to be the case amongst the first PCPs to join and not those participating in the study. Also, the PCPs involved in the study differed from those not participating, which may explain why the hospitalisation rates in both the case and control groups were substantially lower than those for the province as a whole.

Salary versus FFS

The Hickson study was a small trial comparing salaried and FFS paediatricians in the United States.[25] The authors undertook the study because of the increasing shift in the US at that time (1987) towards replacing FFS payment with a salary. The study was carried out in an academic setting: a "resident continuity clinic", which the authors argue is a similar setting to private practice in terms of responsibility for care and the length and nature of relationships with peers and patients. Nine resident paediatricians were randomised to the salary group and nine to FFS payment. The FFS group were paid a fee for each consultation, so the authors' hypothesised that compared with those on salaries, FFS physicians would "attend a greater percentage of their patients' visits, encourage more necessary and unnecessary visits per patient and promote greater loyalty among patients and parents by increasing satisfaction".

Because of the small numbers the study groups were not balanced, in that there were more physicians with an interest in private practice in the salaried group. The authors adjusted their results in the light of this finding and found that the percentage of patient visits attended by the patient's primary physician (continuity of care) was lower in the salaried compared with the FFS group. Salaried PCPs provided fewer necessary and unnecessary well child visits per enrolled patient compared with FFS PCPs. Salaried PCPs appeared to send more patients for emergency visits compared with FFS PCPs, who had an economic incentive to treat their own patients. Unexpectedly though, patients of salaried PCPs appeared to be more satisfied with the access to their physician.

Target payment versus FFS

There is little in the theoretical economic literature about the potential effect of target payments. Economists in the UK have suggested that PCPs might only provide the target level of service and no more, or they may not provide any care at all if they believe they cannot achieve the service target.[26] The introduction of target payments to boost immunisation rates was evaluated in two studies.

Kouides *et al*[27] carried out a trial within the Medicare Influenza Vaccine Demonstration Project in New York, USA between 1991 and 1992. The policy goal of the Project was to determine the cost-effectiveness of making influenza immunisation a covered benefit for Medicare beneficiaries in order to reduce cost as a barrier to increasing immunisation rates amongst elderly patients. PCPs participating in this project received free demonstration vaccines, an $8 administration fee for each Medicare patient they immunised, and used a poster method to track immunisation rates. PCPs randomised to the intervention group received an additional 10 or 20% reimbursement ($0·80 or $1·6 per immunisation) if they immunised 70 or 85% respectively of their eligible population.

PCPs receiving the target payments had an immunisation rate 5·9% higher than the control group, but the difference was not statistically significant. The difference in absolute change from baseline between the intervention and control groups was 6·8%, which was statistically significant. Regression analysis indicated that being in the intervention group and having a lower baseline immunisation rate were, independently, significant predictors of higher immunisation rates.[27] Finally, the authors estimated that the additional cost per extra immunisation gained using target payments was $3·02.

In 1990, the UK government replaced fees for each child immunised with a lump sum payment made if a practice achieved either of two target percentages of eligible children immunised in the practice population (70 and 90%). The assumption made by the government was that a greater economic incentive would increase immunisation rates. Ritchie *et al* examined whether this policy objective had been achieved.[28] The authors calculated immunisation rates for 2- and 5-year-old children registered with 313 GPs in 95 general practices in the Grampian region of Scotland. Fitting immunisation rates using logistic regression, the authors concluded that the steady improvement in these rates over time could not be attributed to the introduction of target payments but to other factors such as better educational materials for health care professionals, information systems and the stimulation of parental knowledge.

The studies described in this section represent the "best" available evidence on the effects of payment systems in primary care. Significant gaps were identified in the evidence base as defined by our inclusion criteria. It was found that there were no studies measuring clinical outcomes and few estimating costs, which precludes any attempts to answer cost-effectiveness questions. There were also no comparisons of salary versus capitation payment. The heterogeneity of practice settings studied and the specific contexts into which the intervention was introduced and its aims also varied widely. In some of the studies there was a lack of evidence that the activities being encouraged or discouraged by the change in payment system were "worthwhile". As a result one should question the usefulness of this evidence base and particularly the generalisability of the findings reviewed. In addition there are doubts about the internal validity of so-called "robust" study designs in the area of doctor payment systems.

Systematic reviews of financial interventions: limitations of the evidence base

How then can "firm knowledge" be established based on the six studies (of which three were randomised trials)? Our position is that this is not possible because of methodological problems inherent in studying health care provider behaviour. The six studies represent a very selected sample (chosen on the basis of design and quality) of the universe of studies in the field. Have the six studies arrived at more valid conclusions than other published studies because only selected designs were included? When, for example, Hickson in the USA found, in an RCT, that doctors on FFS provided more consultations than those on salary, while an observational study in Norway found little evidence of this,[29] are the study findings from Norway invalid? In the following, the issue of whether observational studies always yield less valid results than randomised trials is discussed.

Internal validity

The results of a study are internally valid if they provide unbiased estimates of the parameters for the population from which the sample is drawn. In other words, internal validity is a question of generalising from the sample to the population from which it was drawn. The internal validity may be threatened by confounding as well as selection bias and information bias.[30] Definitions of these phenomena are presented in the glossary.

RCTs are assumed to generate more internally valid results than observational studies because a well-designed and conducted RCT will prevent bias and confounding. In studies of payment systems, and provider behaviour in general, this may not be the case. First, blinding of the study subjects is not possible simply because people cannot react to financial incentives unless they are informed about them. Secondly, once they are informed and they are not happy with their allocation, then they may suffer demoralisation leading to baseline imbalance.[10] Even if there are not baseline imbalances, doctors may change their behaviour either deliberately or unconsciously to influence data collected either by direct observation or by themselves, as many studies of payment systems rely on doctors' own records or reports. Physician preferences are a particular problem in small trials. In the Hickson study,[25] the majority of those allocated to salary payment planned to establish private practice after specialty training and were likely to have preferences for fee-for-service payment. This may have biased the results even though the direction of potential bias is unclear. If, for example, doctors on salary worked slowly because they disliked the payment system, this might exaggerate the difference between the two payment systems. The effect might be opposite if those on salary worked hard because they in general had a preference for hard work (and FFS). Similar effects have been observed in evaluations of organisational interventions.[31]

Selection bias may be an issue in RCTs in which patients, and not doctors, have been allocated to different systems for paying the doctors (two potentially useful RCTs were excluded due to this reason). Randomising patients makes sure that *patient* characteristics cannot explain differences between doctors on different payment systems, but different *doctor* characteristics could still explain differences. The reason is simply that different doctors may have different preferences for payment systems, and doctors on one system are unlikely to be similar to doctors on another system because of self-selection. Randomising doctors avoids this problem but the reasons for choosing the patient as unit of allocation in some trials could have been that they were not designed to test hypotheses about the effects of different payment systems on doctor behaviour. Even if they were, practical or political obstacles may have prevented the trial designers from allocating doctors to different types of payment methods.

External validity

External validity can be defined as the extent to which findings from one population may be generalised to other populations. In other words, if the results of a study are internally valid, do the results apply to other populations? Large proportions of epidemiology textbooks are devoted to methods to ensure internal validity while little is said about external validity. Kleinbaum *et al* state that "concerns about external validity do not lend themselves to quantification and will not be addressed".[30] Rothman devotes one single page to the theme,[32] and underscores that external validity is much more than using statistical methods to ascertain that the findings of a sample can be generalised. Rather, he claims that in most sciences, the process of synthesising knowledge involves "moving from the particulars of a set of observations to the abstraction of a scientific hypothesis or theory that is more or less divorced from time or space". No criteria for establishing external validity are proposed, but the process is described as cumbersome and time-consuming.

Biomedical research focuses on phenomena that are likely to be relatively stable in time and geography. If, for example, studies show that cholesterol-lowering pharmaceuticals are effective in preventing heart attack in Sweden and Scotland, it is reasonable to believe this will be the case in China or the USA as well. When studies of a biomedical phenomenon yield very different results, the tendency is to assume that flaws in some of the studies rather than variation in the phenomenon cause the differences.

In the social sciences, including economics, the study phenomena are likely to be unstable in time and geography. With respect to studies of the effects of payment systems on doctor behaviour, it is conceivable that valid results from one country may not apply to other countries. Unfortunately, because there are no formal tests available, the judgement of external validity has to be based on discretion.

An interesting consequence of the assumed lower *external* validity of social science studies compared with biomedical studies appears to be that *internal* validity has been of less concern to social scientists than to biomedical scientists. When biomedical scientists observe different results from one study to another, it can be interpreted as an indication of potential flaws in some or all of the studies. This would then lead to the pursuit of better study designs. In fact, the increased emphasis of randomised designs can be seen in this perspective. In contrast, social scientists may ascribe differing study results to low external validity. The consequence may be less focus on internal validity.

Is there a role for observational studies in systematic reviews of health policy interventions?

There is little doubt that policy makers would like to see studies with excellent internal validity. However, because of the methodological limitations of RCTs in the area of provider behaviour and because of potential political and practical design issues intrinsic to RCTs in this area, it is unlikely that a great number of them will be seen. Feinstein argues that "investigators who want to get scientific answers to important *clinical* [authors' emphasis] questions will have to reach beyond the constraints of the paradigm that requires formal experimentation as the sole method of science".[33] This position could equally apply to research on payment systems and other health policy issues. Here the term RCT is meant to refer to a design in which exposure to the factor of interest is decided by the experimenter through a random procedure. In principle, confounding variables will then be equally distributed in the groups. When health authorities decide to switch from one payment system to another, this represents a kind of natural experiment. Even though health authorities plan such reforms, they may appear as an unplanned event to doctors. If other factors such as patient and doctor characteristics do not change with the reform, confounding may be less likely. To account for possible time trends, such studies should have several observations before and after the event. Three such studies were included but none of them had as many observations points as one would wish.

The observational study is simply a comparison between two groups at one point in time (cross-sectional study) or observation over time of one or more groups exposed to some factor. In observational studies, differences between groups (for example providers on different payment systems) are adjusted for confounding factors such as patient, doctor and organisation factors. Controlled before and after studies and interrupted time series analysis are used when exposure to specific payment systems is not decided through randomisation but rather "natural" experiments or other events.

During the review process about 330 papers were identified on PCP payment systems. Twenty-six papers had one of the three study designs that were of interest (subsequently 16 were excluded), but approximately twice this number of papers reported observational studies. These studies were not included in the review because appropriate criteria to judge their methodological quality were not readily available. There may also be problems in systematically identifying this type of study in bibliographic sources. If more is to be made of this type of study, we need to be able to understand the methodological shortcomings that can make them inappropriate for health policy and develop methods for identifying them in the literature.

There is ample evidence that confounding and bias may affect observational studies. Proponents of evidence-based medicine argue that RCTs are the gold standard and discourage use of observational studies.[34] Indeed, there is some evidence that observational studies may overestimate effect sizes compared with RCTs.[35] A recent example is a randomised trial of oestrogens for the prevention of heart attack in postmenopausal women.[36] Several observational studies have shown that oestrogens prevent heart attack, while the randomised trial found no effect.

In recent years, however, in the light of new evidence the arguments for ignoring observational study designs have weakened. RCTs may be very selected in terms of their study populations and consequently have limited generalisability.[37] Also, recent studies indicate that well-conducted observational studies yield similar results to RCTs.[38–40] Several systematic attempts have found that in the biomedical area there is no obvious association between the size of the effect and whether the design is experimental or observational.[37,41] These studies have concluded, however, that the outcome of non-randomised studies best approximates the results of RCTs when both use the same inclusion and exclusion criteria[37] and adequately adjust for confounding factors.[41]

Where observational and experimental studies arrive at different conclusions we wish to know whether this is due to lack of internal or external validity. Discrepancies between the good observational studies and randomised trials may be due to low internal validity of the observational studies or low external validity of the trials. For example, the results of observational studies carried out in Norway may differ from those carried out in another country because doctors in these countries react differently to incentives, due to cultural or organisational differences, rather than because the observational studies are badly designed.

If observational studies are to be incorporated into systematic reviews it is important to assess their methodological quality using appropriate criteria. In addition to the usual problems related to selection bias, information bias and confounding, there are three issues that may be of special importance in the area of doctors' payment mechanisms. First, the strongest determinants of doctors' clinical decision making have, in many studies, been patient characteristics. Whether this is because doctors are genuinely altruistic, are governed by medical ethics or medical practice guidelines, or simply comply with patients' wishes and needs for selfish reasons is unknown. The key issue is that doctors appear – not surprisingly – to comply with patients' needs. If observational studies do not include patient characteristics such as age, sex, diagnoses etc., these factors could confound the effect of payment system if there were a statistical association between payment system and the factors. Secondly, doctor characteristics such as age, sex and education, and organisational factors such as doctor density may influence clinical practice and should be accounted for to avoid confounding. Thirdly, studies of payment systems frequently have explanatory variables at different levels in a hierarchical structure (patient, doctor and organisational characteristics). One solution then is to aggregate data and analyse them with the practice as the unit of analysis. However, this would imply a loss of information in the aggregation process. A simpler way would be to keep the patient as the unit of analysis, and use doctor and organisational factors as if they were patient characteristics. This would, however, bias the effect estimates and especially their confidence intervals.[42] The correct method would be to apply hierarchical modelling, but this is unfortunately not always done. A study conducted by one of the authors (ISK) demonstrates the need for hierarchical modelling. The initial publication based on standard regression modelling concluded that doctors on FFS order more laboratory tests than those on salary,[43] while a later analysis with hierarchical modelling did not indicate any significant effect.[44]

Lacking detailed data, some studies have used aggregate register data on doctors' practice to detect differences between doctors' mode of practice. This, however, makes it difficult to adjust for patient and sometimes doctor characteristics, and may introduce the so-called ecological fallacy. The classic example is race and illiteracy in the USA.[45] Robinson observed a relatively strong correlation between the proportion of black people and the proportion of illiterates in the states of the USA. This was because states that had many black people also had many illiterates. There was almost no association between race and illiteracy at the individual level (that is, in the individual state, the risk of being illiterate was independent of race). Similar mistaken inferences may be drawn when using aggregate data to study association between payment system and provider practice.

Concluding remarks

Health care policy makers need to exploit the evidence base or to commission new evaluations if their decisions are to be based, at least partially, on fact rather than beliefs. In making reviews, there are no arguments in favour of being non-systematic rather than systematic. However, systematic reviews may only be of use to policy makers if the appraised evidence is of sufficient quality. The experience related here, of carrying out two systematic reviews of primary care doctor payment systems, gives reasons to doubt that this may be the case in this research area. Indeed, even study designs considered to be "robust" in biomedical research may face methodological limitations when applied to evaluations of payment systems. Therefore, the argument for excluding observational studies from systematic reviews, for example, is not convincing.

Recommendations have also been suggested for improving future evaluations of payment systems, and the need for explicit criteria to assess the methodological quality of observational studies has been highlighted. Whatever their design, studies may be better reported than is currently the case, and authors should be more explicit about the nature of the financial incentives faced by the health care providers. Practice may change slowly when incentives are changed, and the length of follow up and the number of data points should account for this. Only by encouraging further evaluation of payment systems and empirical work on the impact of different study designs can systematic reviews fulfil their potential in this area.

Summary points

- Doctors may be influenced by the way they are paid, but the evidence from high quality studies is fairly limited, and the effects are fairly weak.
- Experimental (randomised) studies may not provide better evidence than observational studies because doctors cannot be blinded to payment system, and may then behave strategically in order to get study results that they prefer.
- The external validity of studies (generalisability) is difficult to judge. This means that results that are true for one country or one health care system, may not be true for others.

Appendix

Characteristics and results of included studies.

Study	Methods	Participants	Interventions	Outcomes	Results
Davidson *et al* 1992[12] (United States)	RCT QUALITY ASSESSMENT Allocation concealed: NOT CLEAR Follow up of PCPs: NOT CLEAR Blinded assessment of outcomes: NOT CLEAR Baseline measurement of outcomes: YES Reliable outcomes: NOT CLEAR Protection against contamination: NOT CLEAR Unit of analysis error	80 PCPs 3770 children aged 18 and below	PCPs in intervention group 1 were paid age-adjusted capitation fees and were at risk for deficits on referral budget but received income for surpluses PCPs in intervention group 2 were paid fees approximately double those in control group for comprehensive examinations (including treatment), routine office visits, initial and follow up hospital visits. Fees were set at levels designed to deliver similar income as group 1 Control group paid lower fees than group 2 for same services	Average number per year per patient (a) 6 months before and (b) during study in: (1) primary care physician visits (2) non-primary care physician visits (3) health and emergency department visits (4) hospitalisations Per cent compliance with CHAP[a] guidelines for: (i) number of PCP visits; and (ii) PCP and outpatient clinic visits over a one year period for children aged: (5) 0–12 months (CHAP = 5) (6) 13–24 months (CHAP = 3) (7) 25–36 months (CHAP = 2) (8) 3–5 years (CHAP = 1) Logistic regression adjusted for higher 6 months utilisation and patient characteristics	Absolute changes – difference between intervention and control (– = intervention lower than control): (1) Capn (a) +0·22; (b) +0·59 ($p \leq 0·05$) FFS (a) +0·77 ($p \leq 0·01$); (b) +0·92 ($p \leq 0·01$) (2) Capn (a) −0·24 ($p \leq 0·01$); (b) −0·25 ($p \leq 0·01$) FFS: (a) −0·03; (b) −0·03 (3) Capn (a) −0·08; (b) −0·32 ($p \leq 0·01$) FFS: (a) −0·24; (b) −0·31 ($p \leq 0·01$) (4) Capn (a) −0·02; (b) −0·02 ($p \leq 0·05$) FFS: (a) −0·04; (b) +0·01 (5) Capn (i) +0·39; (ii) +0·04 FFS (i) +0·56 ($p \leq 0·05$); (ii) +0·10 (6) Capn (i) +0·31; (ii) +0·05 FFS (i) +0·80 ($p \leq 0·05$); (ii) +0·50 ($p \leq 0·05$) (7) Capn (i) +0·55 ($p \leq 0·05$); (ii) +0·22 FFS (i) +0·68 ($p \leq 0·05$); (ii) +0·47 (8) Capn (i) +0·64 ($p \leq 0·05$); (ii) +0·18 FFS (i) +1·00 ($p \leq 0·05$); (ii) +0·58 ($p \leq 0·05$)

[a]CHAP, New York's Child Health Assurance Program periodicity schedule, based on the AAP Guidelines for Health Supervision.

(Continued)

Study	Methods	Participants	Interventions	Outcomes	Results
Krasnik *et al* 1990[19] (Denmark)	CBA QUALITY ASSESSMENT Similar control site: NOT CLEAR Follow up of PCPs: NOT CLEAR Blinded assessment of outcomes: NO Baseline measurement of outcomes: YES Reliable outcomes: NO Protection against contamination: YES	100 GPs in Copenhagen City (Denmark) were selected at random as the study group 326 control group GPs in Copenhagen county	GPs in Copenhagen City paid by capitation prior to October 1987 and FFS in combination with capitation after Fees paid for face-to-face, telephone and home visit consultations, repeat prescriptions, 40 special services (e.g. cervical smear tests), 40 laboratory investigations (e.g. haemoglobin concentration), and preventive services (e.g. immunisations) GPs in control group paid by mix of FFS/capitation throughout study	Differences between six months before intervention and (a) 6 and (b) 12 months after in the following outcomes over a 1 week period per 1000 patients: (1) Face-to-face consultations (including home visits) (2) Telephone consultations (3) Renewal of prescription (4) Diagnostic services (5) Curative services (6) Referrals to specialists (7) Referrals to hospital	Absolute changes – difference between intervention and control (– = intervention lower than control): (1) (a) +7·2 ($p \leq 0·05$); (b) −0·5 (2) (a) +10·2 ($p \leq 0·05$); (b) +11 ($p \leq 0·05$) (3) (a) −9; (b) −27·4 ($p \leq 0·05$) (4) (a) +32·8 ($p \leq 0·05$); (b) +52·2 ($p \leq 0·05$) (5) (a) +88·6 ($p \leq 0·05$); (b) +79·8 ($p \leq 0·05$) (6) (a) −9·3; (b) −21·2 ($p \leq 0·05$) (7) (a) −9·7; (b) −33·7 ($p \leq 0·05$)
Hutchison *et al* 1994 (Canada)	CBA QUALITY ASSESSMENT Control site similar: YES Follow up of PCPs: YES Blinded assessment of outcomes: YES Baseline measurement of outcomes: YES Reliable outcomes: YES Protection against contamination: YES	39 PCPs in intervention group and 77 in control (Ontario, Canada)	Intervention: PCPs changed their payment from FFS to a mix of capitation and an ambulatory incentive payment where the health service organisation received a payment if their hospitalisation rate was lower than the regional rate Control: FFS	(1) Hospital separations (admissions) (2) Hospital days Outcomes expressed as differences in age, sex and social assistance adjusted rates per 1000 patients between one year before intervention and three years after	Absolute difference between intervention and control (– = intervention lower than control): (1) −0·2 ($p = 0·312$) (2) +3 ($p = 0·774$)

Continued

(Continued)

Study	Methods	Participants	Interventions	Outcomes	Results
Hickson *et al* 1987[25] (United States)	RCT QUALITY ASSESSMENT Allocation concealed: YES Follow up of PCPs: NOT CLEAR Blinded assessment of outcomes: NOT CLEAR Baseline measurement of outcomes: NOT CLEAR Reliable outcomes: NOT CLEAR Protection against contamination: NO No unit of analysis error	10 second year and 8 third year paediatric residents (USA)	Intervention group paid by salary Control group paid $2 per visit	Average number (over a 9 month period) per PCP of: (1) Patient visits attended (2) Patients enrolled Per enrolled patient: (3) Emergency room visits (4) Scheduled visits (5) Completed visits (6) Sick, primary visits (7) Sick follow up visits (8) Well child visits (9) Per cent of visits attended by patient's primary physician (continuity) (10) Compliance with American Academy of Pediatrics' guidelines: (i) Per cent of recommended visits missed (ii) Per cent of visits in excess of the recommended (11) Patient satisfaction (i) Humanness (ii) Continuity/convenience (iii) Access to physician (iv) Overall satisfaction	Absolute difference between intervention and control (– = intervention lower than control): (1) –6·8 (2) +11·7 ($p \leq 0·05$)** (3) +10 ($p \leq 0·05$) (4) –0·86 ($p \leq 0·05$) (5) –0·49 ($p \leq 0·05$) (6) +0·03 (7) –0·09 (8) –0·43 ($p \leq 0·05$) (9) –8·3 ($p \leq 0·05$) (10) (i) +6·4 ($p \leq 0·05$); (ii) –13·3 ($p \leq 0·05$) (11) Patient satisfaction: (i) humanness (ns); (ii) continuity/convenience (ns); (iii) access to physician: higher in salary ($p \leq 0·05$); (iv) overall satisfaction (ns)
Kouides *et al* 1998[27] (United States)	RCT QUALITY ASSESSMENT Allocation	27 practices in the intervention group 27 in the control group	PCPs in intervention group received a fee and an additional 10% ($0·8) or 20% ($1·6) reimbursement per shot according to whether they	(1) Mean influenza vaccination rate in the intervention period (1991) (2) Change in influenza vaccination rate from	Absolute difference between intervention and control (– = intervention lower than control): (1) +5·9% (68·6% in intervention group; 62·7% in the control

Continued

(Continued)

Study	Methods	Participants	Interventions	Outcomes	Results
	concealed: NOT CLEAR Follow up of PCPs: YES Blinded assessment of primary outcome: YES Baseline measurement of outcomes: YES Reliable outcomes: NOT CLEAR Protection against contamination: YES Unit of analysis error for one of the outcomes (overall immunisation rate)	(New York, USA) 21196 nursing home patients in intervention group and 17 608 in control group	immunised 70% or 85% (respectively) of the eligible population Control group PCPs received the $8 fee only	baseline year (between 1991 and 1990) (3) Overall influenza vaccination rate – sum of all immunisation given divided by the sum of eligible patients – in the intervention period (1991)	group); $p = 0{\cdot}22$ (2) +6·8% (10·3% in intervention group; 3·5% in the control group) $p = 0{\cdot}03$ (3) +6·8% (66·9% in intervention group; 60·1% in the control group) p = N/A
Ritchie *et al* 1992[28] (United Kingdom (Scotland))	ITS QUALITY ASSESSMENT Protection against secular changes: YES Sufficient data points to enable reliable statistical inference: NOT DONE Formal test for trend: YES Data collection identical before and after the intervention: YES Intervention unlikely to affect data collection: YES Blinded assessment of primary outcome: YES Completeness of data set: YES Reliability of outcome measure: YES	95 general practices (313 GPs) (Scotland, UK) Children	PCPs previously paid a fee for childhood immunisations after 1990 received a lower or higher payment according to whether they immunised 70% or 90% (respectively) of the eligible population	Changes over a 20 month period (January 1990 to September 1991) in the number of practices achieving at least: (1) 95% primary immunisation rates (2) 90% primary immunisation rates (3) 95% pre-school immunisation rates (4) 90% pre-school immunisation rates (5) Proportion of immunisations given by PCPs	Absolute difference between intervention and control (– = intervention lower than control): (1) +49·5% (from 31% to 80%) (2) +18·9% (from 73% to 92%) (3) +41·1% (from 23% to 64%) (4) +42·1% (from 38% to 80%) (5) +12% (from 86% to 98%) Authors fitted the trend in immunisations using a logistic regression model and found that there was no evidence that the overall linear trend had changed as a result of the introduction of target payments

** No significant difference when authors adjusted for differential interest in private practice.

References

1 Mulrow CD. Rationale for systematic reviews. *BMJ* 1994;**309**:597–9.

2 Ham C, Hunter DJ, Robinson R. Evidence based policymaking. *BMJ* 1995;**310**:71–2.

3 Florin D. Barriers to evidence based policy. *BMJ* 1996;**313**:894–5.

4 Gaynor M. Issues in the Industrial Organization of the Market for Physician Services. *J Econ Manage Strat* 1994;**3**:211–55.

5 McGuire T. Physician agency. In: Culyer A, Newhouse J, eds. *Handbook of Health Economics.* Amsterdam: Elsevier Science, 2000, pp. 461–536.

6 Bero L, Grilli R, Grimshaw J, Mowatt G, Oxman AD, Zwarenstein M. The Cochrane Effective Practice and Organisation of Care Group (EPOC) Module. *The Cochrane Database of Systematic Reviews.* Oxford: Update Software, 2000.

7 Giuffrida A, Gosden T, Forland F, Kristiansen IS, Sergison M, Leese B, Pedersen L, Sutton M. Target payments in primary care: effects on professional practice and health care outcomes (Cochrane Review). *The Cochrane Library,* Issue 3. Oxford: Update Software, 2000.

8 Gosden T, Forland F, Kristiansen IS, Sutton M, Leese B, Giuffrida A, Sergison M, Pedersen L. Capitation, salary, fee-for-service and mixed systems of payment: effects on the behaviour of primary care physicians (Cochrane Review). *The Cochrane Library,* Issue 3. Oxford: Update Software, 2001.

9 Gosden T, Forland F, Kristiansen IS, Sutton M, Leese B, Giuffrida A *et al.* Impact of payment method on behaviour of primary care physicians: a systematic review. *J Health Serv Res Policy* 2001;**6**:44–55.

10 Cook T, Campbell D. *Quasi-experimentation. Design and analysis issues for field settings.* Chicago: Rand McNally, 1979.

11 Hohlen MM, Manheim LM, Fleming GV, Davidson SM, Yudkowsky BK, Werner SM *et al.* Access to office-based physicians under capitation reimbursement and Medicaid case management. Findings from the Children's Medicaid Program. *Med Care* 1990;**28**:59–68.

12 Davidson SM, Manheim LM, Werner SM, Hohlen MM, Yudkowsky BK, Fleming GV. Prepayment with office-based physicians in publicly funded programs: results from the Children's Medicaid Program. *Pediatrics* 1992;**89**:761–7.

13 Pontes MC. Agency theory: a framework for analyzing physician services. *Health Care Manage Rev* 1995;**20**:57–67.

14 Lerner C, Claxton K. *Modelling the behaviour of general practitioners. A theoretical foundation for studies of fundholding.* Centre for Health Economics, University of York, 1994.

15 McGuire TG, Pauly MV. Physician response to fee changes with multiple payers. *J Health Econ* 1991;**10**:385–410.

16 Yett DE, Der W, Ernst RL, Hay JW. Physician pricing and health insurance reimbursement. *Health Care Financ Rev* 1983;**5**:69–80.

17 Flierman HA, Groenewegen PP. Introducing fees for services with professional uncertainty. *Health Care Financ Rev* 1992;**14**:107–15.

18 Krasnik A, Gottschau A. Doctor and patient characteristics as modifiers of the effect of a changing remuneration system in general practice. *Dan Med Bull* 1993;**40**:380–2.

19 Krasnik A, Groenewegen PP, Pedersen PA, von Scholten P, Mooney G, Gottschau A *et al.* Changing remuneration systems: effects on activity in general practice. *BMJ* 1990;**300**:1698–701.

20 Rice TH. The impact of changing medicare reimbursement rates on physician-induced demand. *Med Care* 1983;**21**:803–15.

21 Evans RG. Supplier induced demand: some empirical evidence and implications. In: Perlman M, ed. *The economics of health and medical care.* New York: Wiley, 1974, pp. 162–73.

22 Donaldson C, Gerard K. Paying general practitioners: shedding light on the review of health services. *J R Coll Gen Pract* 1989;**39**:114–17.

23 Hughes D, Yule B. The effect of per-item fees on the behaviour of general practitioners. *J Health Econ* 1992;**11**:413–37.

24 Hutchison B, Birch S, Hurley J, Lomas J, Stratford-Devai F. Do physician-payment mechanisms affect hospital utilization? A study of Health Service Organizations in Ontario. *CMAJ* 1996;**154**:653–61.

25 Hickson GB, Altemeier WA, Perrin JM. Physician reimbursement by salary or fee-for-service: effect on physician practice behavior in a randomized prospective study. *Pediatrics* 1987;**80**:344–50.
26 Hughes D. General practitioners and the new contract: promoting better health through financial incentives. *Health Policy* 1993;**25**:39–50.
27 Kouides RW, Bennett NM, Lewis B, Cappuccio JD, Barker WH, LaForce FM. Performance-based physician reimbursement and influenza immunization rates in the elderly. The Primary-Care Physicians of Monroe County. *Am J Prev Med* 1998; **14**:89–95.
28 Ritchie LD, Bisset AF, Russell D, Leslie V, Thomson I. Primary and preschool immunisation in Grampian: progress and the 1990 contract. *BMJ* 1992;**304**:816–19.
29 Kristiansen IS, Mooney G. The general practitioner's use of time: is it influenced by the remuneration system? *Soc Sci Med* 1993;**37**:393–9.
30 Kleinbaum D, Kupper L, Morgenstern H. *Epidemiologic research*. New York: Van Nostrand Reinhold, 1982.
31 Saretsky G. The OEO PC experiment and the John Henry effect. *Phi Delta Kappan* 1972;**53**:579–81.
32 Rothman K, Greenland S. *Modern epidemiology*. Philadelphia: Lippincott–Raven, 1998.
33 Feinstein AR. An additional basic science for clinical medicine: II. The limitations of randomized trials. *Ann Intern Med* 1983;**99**:544–50.
34 British Medical Association. *Medical ethics today*. London: BMA, 1993.
35 Sacks H, Chalmers TC, Smith H, Jr. Randomized versus historical controls for clinical trials. *Am J Med* 1982;**72**:233–40.
36 Hulley S, Grady D, Bush T, Furberg C, Herrington D, Riggs B *et al*. Randomized trial of estrogen plus progestin for secondary prevention of coronary heart disease in postmenopausal women. Heart and Estrogen/progestin Replacement Study (HERS) Research Group. *JAMA* 1998;**280**:605–13.
37 Britton A, McKee M, Black N, McPherson K, Sanderson C, Bain C. Choosing between randomised and non-randomised studies: a systematic review. *Health Technol Assess* 1998;**2**:i–124.
38 McKee M, Britton A, Black N, McPherson K, Sanderson C, Bain C. Methods in health services research. Interpreting the evidence: choosing between randomised and non-randomised studies. *BMJ* 1999;**319**:312–15.
39 Benson K, Hartz AJ. A comparison of observational studies and randomized, controlled trials. *N Engl J Med* 2000;**342**:1878–86.
40 Concato J, Shah N, Horwitz RI. Randomized, controlled trials, observational studies, and the hierarchy of research designs. *N Engl J Med* 2000;**342**:1887–92.
41 MacLehose RR, Reeves BC, Harvey IM, Sheldon TA, Russell IT, Black AM. A systematic review of comparisons of effect sizes derived from randomised and non-randomised studies. *Health Technol Assess* 2000;**4**:1–154.
42 Rice N, Leyland A. Multilevel models: applications to health data. *J Health Serv Res Policy* 1996;**1**:154–64.
43 Kristiansen IS, Hjortdahl P. The general practitioner and laboratory utilization: why does it vary? *Fam Pract* 1992;**9**:22–7.
44 Kristiansen IS. *Factors affecting doctors' decision making*. Thesis, Institute of Community Medicine, University of Tromso, Norway, 1996.
45 Robinson W. Ecological correlations and the behaviour of individuals. *Am Socio Rev* 1950;**15**:351–7.

10: Making the problem fit the solution: evidence-based decision making and "Dolly" economics

STEPHEN BIRCH

Introduction

Evidence-based decision making is a normative approach to decision making in health care under which decisions should involve the "conscientious, explicit and judicious use of current best evidence".[1] Associated with this approach, increased interest has emerged in systematic reviews of research studies (application of explicit criteria to the identification and review of individual studies) and meta-analyses of research (the application of statistical principles to pooling results from different studies of similar interventions). The Cochrane Collaboration provides an international context for gathering, analysing and disseminating the findings of these activities.[2] Together these initiatives share the common goal of improving the quality of the information on health care effectiveness available to decision makers.

The evidence-based approach in health care emerged from the interests of clinical epidemiologists,[3,4] and has since spread to health services research and health policy.[5,6] However, the underlying rationale of the approach is consistent with the three fundamental concepts of economics: *scarcity, choice* and *opportunity cost*. Ageing populations, technological developments in health care and increasing public expectations all lead to increasing demands on the resources made available to health care services. Hence health care resources are increasingly *scarce*. The political and fiscal climates of the late twentieth century highlighted the importance of *choices* in response to increasing scarcity. Increasing expenditure on health care is viewed in many countries as neither a solution nor even an option for responding to this problem. It has not worked in the past, and the fiscal consequences may not be supported by electorates. Instead, attention has focused on considering what is achieved by the current practices and whether different practices would achieve more – essentially a matter of *opportunity costs*. Clinical epidemiology focuses on what can be achieved (effectiveness) without comparing this to what has to be forgone (efficiency). As a result, economists participate in the evidence-based movement in order to inject some "resource" context into what is primarily a clinical epidemiology exercise.[7] However the role of economists has been largely confined to adding economic components to the evidence-based approach and has not extended to considering the appropriateness of the evidence-based approach from an economics perspective.

In this chapter the methods followed in the evidence-based approach are shown to emerge from a particular scientific paradigm which is generally not compatible with either an economics (or, more generally, social sciences) way of thinking or with the needs of decision makers. As a result, the incorporation of economics in the evidence-based approach involves "cloning" the non-economics scientific paradigm for economics. Decision makers are left to address problems using the research generated under this narrow paradigm. However, decisions based on the findings from these studies can be associated with reductions in the efficiency of use of health care resources and increasing inequalities in health. As an alternative, research could be based on a broader scientific paradigm in order to better serve the needs of decision makers. Information is identified to supplement the existing research "evidence" for the purposes of decision making as a first step towards a problem-centred approach to informed decision making.

Scientific paradigms, policy-informing research and "Dolly" economics

The evidence-based approach is based on the premise that the findings of high quality research studies ought to be useful to, and hence used by, decision makers.[8] As a consequence, considerable resources have been devoted to the timely dissemination of research to decision makers and facilitation of the use of research findings in the decision making process. In this way the evidence-based approach is "research-led" and "intervention-focused" – researchers providing information about interventions that decision makers "should" use based on the assumption that the interests of the researchers satisfy the needs of the decision makers.[9] However, in the research environment of clinical epidemiologists, as well as of health services researchers and health economists with whom they collaborate, attention is focused on (or even confined to) the relationship between exposure to an intervention and responsiveness, in terms of health status changes among a population with a particular clinical condition. The (implicit) question asked by the researcher is "*does this intervention work on average, in this population*?". Other possible explanations of observed changes in health status confound or confuse the estimation of the intervention–outcome relationship. By excluding certain types of individuals from the population selected for study and randomising the selected population between those who receive the intervention and those who do not, the probability of observed changes in health status being explained by other factors (or determinants of health) is reduced.

Decision makers do not have the luxury of "cleansing" problems of the context in which they occur. Instead, their needs are "problem-focused"; they need to know "under what conditions will individuals with the condition benefit from this intervention?" and "will the intervention work given the circumstances of the subjects for whom it is being considered?".[10] Abstracting research from reality, although serving the intellectual curiosity of the researcher, fails to serve the needs of the decision maker or subjects. This discrepancy arises from the scientific paradigm underlying the evidence-based approach.[9]

The Newtonian paradigm: The proponents of the evidence-based approach work within a Newtonian paradigm incorporating doctrines of reductionism and universality. **Reductionism** maintains that all knowledge can be broken down into small units. Analysis is therefore based on the disaggregation of problems into smaller parts. Explanations for, and solutions to, these smaller parts then become generalised as solutions to the larger problem. **Universality** assumes the existence of a reality or truth that is consistent and value free, and which is beyond perception. This underlying reality can be discovered by careful application of research methods. Because the collection and analysis of data are postulated to be value free, research uncovers objective facts and separates what is true from what is false. For example, under this paradigm we can study outcomes associated with a health care intervention to establish facts about whether the intervention works or not. Recognition of the complexity of the production of health in populations leads to reductionist modifications in research designs such as the randomised controlled trial to "control" for these potential "confounders".

The Value Critical Systems (VCS) paradigm: The relevance and validity of the Newtonian paradigm for informing decision making concerned with systems such as the production of health in populations is questionable. An alternative "value critical systems" (VCS) paradigm for health research has been proposed that is more consistent with a social sciences approach to guide problem-focused or socially relevant research.[11] The VCS paradigm is based on the doctrines of expansionism, relativity and teleology. Under **expansionism** all problems are subsets of larger problems. Analyses confined to observations of "individual" parts disregard the possible influence of the "bigger picture". To understand the interdependent system, problems must be analysed within the system (the "bigger picture") using integrative thinking. For example, the poor social conditions of unemployed single mothers might be an important part of exploring the problem of smoking among women. Randomisation of women smokers between intervention and control groups simply conceals potentially important factors in understanding the problem as well as identifying effective interventions.

Relativity assumes that truths are contextually determined. For example, we cannot expect to find an answer to the question of whether capitation for physicians is associated with better quality health care. Instead, the effects of capitation on quality of care will depend on a whole range of factors that are specific to the application, including the level of capitation payments, the design of the health care system, the types of physician in question and the population being studied. In this way there is no universal reality.

Teleology contends that systems are inherently purposeful and hence normative. Researchers approach the discovery of even contextually dependent truths with an inherent set of ethics and morals which guide the research process. This may be reflected in the problems we choose to study, the types of questions we ask about these problems or the constructs we choose to measure. Each stage of the research process involves subjective considerations which are determined usually by the values of the researcher, even if these values are sometimes concealed as scientific convention. Five-year survival rates and 95% confidence intervals are two examples of purposeful choices that introduce values into the research study. Whether these values are shared by subjects with the condition is not considered.

These underlying principles of the VCS paradigm are a familiar part of the social sciences, the discipline of economics and much of the field of applied economics. Indeed, major advances have been contributed by more traditional economic thinking in the development and application of a wide range of conceptual frameworks concerning the production of health, illness and recovery in populations.[12,13] However, collaboration with clinical epidemiologists and biostatisticians in the evidence-based movement has been based on the narrow Newtonian scientific paradigm on which these other disciplines are based. Cloning Dolly the sheep was seen by many as a major advance in science. But should cloning be extended to matters of scientific paradigms? It could be argued that the implicit adoption of the Newtonian paradigm by economists involved in the evidence-based movement is simply "Dolly" economics.

The production of health, illness and recovery in populations

Concerns with systematic, persistent and, in many cases, increasing inequalities in health within populations have been associated with the development of broad conceptual frameworks in the social sciences literature for explaining the production and distribution of health, illness and recovery in populations.[13–16] Under these frameworks interest in the utilisation and outcomes of health care is complemented by the recognition of the potential roles of individual-level factors such as income and education as well as the social, cultural, economic and physical environments as determinants of health. Two important economic implications arise from these frameworks.[10] First, demands for health care compete with demands for other health-enhancing activities for society's scarce resources. The provision of health care therefore involves an opportunity cost in terms of other health producing activities forgone. The importance of the measurement and comparison of health outcomes is therefore not confined to health care interventions but extends to choices between health care and non-health care programmes. Second, demands for health improvements, including the protection and promotion of health as well as its restoration, compete for resources with demands for other sources of wellbeing. Making the best use of resources cannot be determined by measurement of health outcomes alone. Instead, the protection, promotion and restoration of health are evaluated in the context of other uses of resources by considering the contribution of health outcomes to overall wellbeing.

Emerging from these frameworks is the notion of multiple pathways to health, illness and recovery involving different "determinants" of health. These pathways do not represent individual and separable "factor determinants" such as health care, income and education. Instead, the pathways represent the interfaces between these different influences on health and wellbeing. For example, the impact of a health care intervention on individuals with a particular health condition (whether it works) may vary according to the socioeconomic circumstances of the individual.[10] So socioeconomic circumstances can influence health through several routes: affecting the risk of illness; affecting uptake or compliance with the intervention; and affecting the outcome of the intervention. The notion of interacting determinants of (or pathways to) health has several important implications for decision making based on "intervention-focused" research.

Concealing underlying causes of problems: A population with the same condition may differ in the underlying causes of the condition. For example, the poor economic circumstances of smokers with low incomes may be part of the cause of the problem of smoking (as well as other problems) and will likely differ from the causes of smoking in non-low income subjects.

Failing to compare "like with like": Interventions aimed at treating the condition (as opposed to underlying causes of the condition) may have systematic differences in outcomes among different social groups.[17–20] Where other "determinants of health" are at "favourable" levels for health, such as the environments to which middle class subjects are exposed, one might expect outcomes of the clinical intervention to be greater than in subjects with "detrimental" levels of other health determinants.

Increasing social inequalities in health: Where information on differences in effectiveness by social group is concealed by "intervention-focused" research, decisions based on this research could increase social inequalities in health. Even where research identifies between-group differences in the effectiveness of an intervention, an evidence-based approach to allocating resources for this intervention would give priority to middle class patients for whom outcomes are greater. This leads to the greatest impact of the use of these resources **for this intervention** within the population. However this focus on **the intervention** as the subject of study as opposed to **the population of subjects with the problem** further increases the inequalities in health within the population.

Constraining the potential effectiveness of resource use: Initiatives aimed at the underlying causes of a condition (for example poor social circumstances) as opposed to interventions for the condition *per se* (for example a drug), have the potential to improve outcomes in multiple ways: by reducing the incidence of this, and potentially other, conditions among the poor; by improving compliance with this, and potentially other, interventions among poor subjects; and by improving effectiveness of this, and potentially other, interventions when provided to these subjects.

As a result, health and social policies need not be seen as rival or competing approaches to the production of health, illness and recovery in populations. On the contrary, the effectiveness of health care interventions and hence the rate of return on investments in these interventions, might be enhanced by social policies that provide a more "receptive" population of subjects for the intervention. The development of policies aimed at combating drug abuse may be a good example of this. But "intervention-focused" research would generally not identify these opportunities and hence fails to serve the best interests of even those researchers concerned exclusively with health care interventions.

Validity and informed decision making

The limitations of intervention-focused research for addressing decision makers' problems can be broadly summarised as twofold; failing to study populations where the problems are greatest (resulting from selection, and leading to a lack of external validity) and failing to study the distribution of costs and consequences in those populations that are studied (leading to a lack of generalisability of conclusions to members of the study sample, or internal validity despite the use of an apparently rigorous design).

To clinical epidemiologists (and those researchers with whom they collaborate) intellectual interest in the intervention's effectiveness *per se*, scientific rigour concerned with excluding confounding explanations, together with scarce resources for research studies mean that evaluations, both clinical and economic, focus attention on a selected group of subjects. As a result, the findings of the evaluation are specific to the group of subjects studied (the study population) and decision makers are left to consider whether these findings are relevant for subjects with the same condition but not part of the selected sample, or for particular individuals within the study population. As Sackett *et al*[21] note, "clinical evidence can inform, but can never replace, individual clinical expertise that decides whether the external evidence applies to the individual patient at all". However, in the absence of other information about this or other interventions in subjects with the condition but excluded from the sample, the temptation is to consider the findings as "better than nothing" or good enough. In other words, external validity may be assumed implicitly by the decision maker, despite the concerns of the researcher, because the researcher has failed to provide the decision maker with information relevant to the problem faced.

Similarly, research is usually designed in a way that is unable to inform the decision makers about particular types of subjects or differences between subjects within the study. These matters of validity and generalisability, both internal and external, give rise to a number of considerations about the conduct of the research study. These include issues concerning sample selection, study design, data analysis and the presentation of findings. In each case, the processes followed in traditional research studies appear to have more to do with the intellectual curiosity or convenience of the researcher as opposed to the needs of the decision maker.

Sample selection

This involves the identification of particular characteristics among subjects for use in excluding these subjects from the study. In some cases this relates to ethical considerations such as subjects for whom inclusion would be harmful given their current condition. However, in many cases the rationale for sample selection has nothing to do with the interests of the subjects and hence is of little if any relevance to addressing the problem at hand. For example, a common exclusion criterion is the inability of subjects to communicate in English. If individuals who do not speak English do not suffer from the condition there is no need for the exclusion criteria. The existence of exclusion criteria means potentially important information for decision makers is not produced – information about whether the factor, in this case language, and factors that might be associated with language (for example, a higher prevalence of poor socioeconomic conditions among non-English speaking immigrants) are correlated with outcomes.

Studying minority language groups and other "hard to reach" populations imposes additional burdens on researchers and those who fund research. However, where decision makers are responsible for the delivery of programmes to entire populations, the use of information based on selected samples, where selection is based on little more than researcher convenience, involves both ethical and scientific considerations. In the context of multiple determinants of the health of populations, it is important that the sample selected for a study of an intervention for a particular condition should reflect the distribution of the condition in the population, and hence the distribution of the many other factors that might affect changes in the condition. Exclusion of subjects on the basis of research convenience involves loss of potentially important information about the intervention in the treatment of the condition in the population.

Randomisation is used in the allocation of study subjects between intervention and control groups as a key element of addressing variations in populations in order to *avoid* bias. The failure to extend randomisation to the selection of subjects from all individuals in a population with the condition (subject to any true ethical exclusions) essentially involves the selection of a biased study sample.

Study design

External validity is about not assuming the findings of a study apply to subjects excluded from the study. Internal validity, on the other hand, relates to ensuring that the findings of the study pertain to the particular subjects included in the study. As described above, random allocation of subjects between intervention and control groups is used to safeguard internal validity, that is, to minimise the risk of confounding in the study. As a result, the researcher does not need to collect information on these potential confounding health determinants. Under random allocations of subjects, the distribution of other health determinants among subjects should be approximately the same in both intervention and control groups. The emphasis behind this methodology is therefore on excluding alternative explanations of the finding as opposed to the value of the finding *per se*. But whose interests are being served by this particular design – the subjects, the decision makers or the researchers? For example, studies provide information on whether the intervention is better than the control, *on average*, in the sample of subjects selected for study.[1] However, population heterogeneity might affect whether the intervention works or not (or how well it works), something that random allocation is designed to conceal. Within both the intervention and control groups there is likely to be a distribution of outcomes (levels of success and failure). But the information to describe this distribution is not usually collected or, if it is, not usually reported. It is little consolation to me (or to people like me, or health care decision makers serving people like me) that I was allocated to the intervention that worked on average if I happened to be one of the subjects who died. If the information were collected (and reported) it might be found that for all the people like me, I was less likely to die without the intervention – presumably important information for decision makers as well as subjects.

Data analysis

The findings of a study, although internally valid for the population studied as a whole, need not apply to all within the study population and hence to particular decisions faced by the decision maker. Results based on comparisons of groups consisting of "different" individuals can therefore suppress potentially important information to decision makers about individuals or subgroups within the selected sample. Where information on the distributions of outcomes within groups is not collected, or where that information is suppressed, decision makers may seek comfort in trying to make the right decision for the population (or that part of it in the study sample) on average. However, concealing the role of other factors can undermine even the internal validity of the research.

Simpson[22] showed that summarising information over groups with different levels of important factors (for example incomes) where the subjects were not randomised to those groups, can lead to paradoxical results. One programme can appear to be more effective than a different programme, based on study findings, when in fact it produces less outcomes from the same resources. Simpson's paradox[23] can be illustrated by the data presented in Tables 10.1 and 10.2. The decision maker is faced with demands to introduce two separate programmes aimed at treating different conditions, A and B, and has to decide which should have priority. Data from randomised clinical trials are made available (Table 10.1). Each trial is based on a sample of 200 subjects randomly allocated to intervention and control groups. Treatment for condition A is associated with a greater incremental outcome (that is, outcomes in those subjects receiving intervention as compared with subjects in the control group) than treatment for condition B. As a result, effectiveness, as measured by the average additional outcome per subject receiving the intervention, is greater for A than for B. For simplicity, assume that the cost of treating 100 patients with condition A is the same as the cost of treating 100 patients with condition B. In that case, based on the evidence of the trials, the decision maker will give priority to the intervention for treating condition A, *ceteris paribus*. Note that the trials did not collect or analyse data concerning other determinants of health. Subjects were selected on the basis of the condition to be treated. Any differences in the study population in other health determinants are dealt with by random allocation of subjects between intervention and control groups.

Suppose the social distribution of conditions A and B in the population differ, with A more prevalent in richer groups (R) and B more prevalent in poorer groups (P). Table 10.2 disaggregates the data from Table 10.1 into rich and poor groups. Note that for both trials randomisation "works" with exactly half of each socioeconomic group randomised to receive the intervention. Both interventions provide positive outcomes for both groups of subjects but effectiveness is greater for R than P for both interventions.

Table 10.1 Randomised controlled trial for interventions for two different conditions.

	Treatment for condition A	Treatment for condition B
Subjects (*N*)	**200**	**200**
Randomised to:		
Intervention	100	100
Control	100	100
Outcomes (QALYs) (Intervention–Control)	**900**	**880**
Effectiveness (QALY/*N*)	**9**	**8·8**

Table 10.2 Randomised controlled trial results by socioeconomic group.

	Treatment for condition A	Treatment for condition B
Subjects (*N*)	**200**	**200**
Of which:		
Group P	40	160
Group R	160	40
Randomised to intervention		
Group P	20	80
Group R	80	20
Outcomes (QALYs)	**900**	**880**
Of which:		
Group P	100	640
Group R	800	240
Effectiveness (QALY/*N*)	**9**	**8·8**
Of which:		
Group P	5	8
Group R	10	12

More important, however, is the comparison of the two interventions within socioeconomic groups. For both R and P the intervention for condition B is more effective than the intervention for condition A. In other words, the findings from the trials imply that the intervention for A is better than the intervention for B even though this is not true for either subgroup. The same paradox can occur where effectiveness is the same for all subjects but the costs of the two interventions differ by socioeconomic group.

The internal validity produced by the randomised controlled trial of an intervention is limited to whether the intervention being studied works (produces greater outcomes and/or lower costs) on average in the sample studied relative to a control. But decisions do not generally concern whether to provide an intervention or the control. Instead, decision makers need to know whether to use resources to serve subjects with a particular condition with one of several interventions or to use the same resources to serve subjects with a different condition using one of several interventions. Such decisions require information on the level of effectiveness, not merely its presence. Simpson's paradox shows that the internal validity of the randomised controlled trial does not extend to the level of effectiveness. Again, the interests of the researchers appear to be dominating the needs of decision makers in the way the results are analysed.

Presentation of findings

Constraints on available research funds are sometimes used to defend existing approaches to research. However, these discussions are less prominent in communications with decision makers, or in those parts of scientific communications that are used by decision makers. As an example, consider the reporting of the NASCET trial of endarterectomy for the treatment of high grade symptomatic carotid stenosis.[24] The authors of the study, based on a well-designed trial by a highly respected and experienced group of investigators, devoted approximately one sixth of the text of the scientific publication to the "special circumstances" of the trial. These circumstances covered the selection of subjects, physicians and centres in which the interventions were performed, factors that might undermine the validity of the findings for different types of subjects, physicians and settings. The structured abstract concludes that "carotid endarterectomy reduced the risk of stroke" without any qualification being given to this finding or any mention being made of the special circumstances of the trial. As a result, these important considerations are likely to escape the attention of a decision maker faced with the difficult decision about whether a programme should be funded, or a physician faced with a decision about what treatment to recommend for a patient with this condition. This tendency to exclude qualifications to the validity of studies from those parts of research reports to which decision makers are more likely to be exposed further undermines the validity of the evidence-based approach from the perspective of health care decision making.

Discussion

The Cochrane database is essentially a collection of answers to questions of interest to members of the collaboration. These questions emerge from members' intellectual curiosity and rarely pay attention to the contexts in which problems occur and are addressed by decision makers. This leaves the decision maker with solutions in search of problems. The central theme of the Cochrane Collaboration concerns establishing the effectiveness of interventions and reflects a clinical epidemiology perspective. However, where economics has been introduced into "evidence-based" decision making, its application has been constrained by this restricted "clinical" perspective. This fails to reflect the complex pathways of the production of health, illness and recovery in populations presented by an economics perspective and faced by decision makers. The use of this information in decision making could be associated with the inefficient use of scarce health care resources as well as increasing social inequalities in health.

Glasziou and Irwig[25] provide an analytical framework for individualising treatment decisions based on two sources of information. Meta-analyses of randomised controlled trials of the interventions under consideration provide information on the change in relative risk and whether this change varies with the baseline risk. Cohort studies provide information on the multiple correlates of risk through the estimation of multivariate risk equations. The decision maker can then predict the outcome and risk of harm for an individual patient. In the examples presented by the authors, the correlates of risk considered are restricted to clinical factors. But the approach would be equally appropriate for non-clinical determinants of health, illness and recovery. Of course, in order to predict outcomes for different social groups, both the randomised trials and the cohort studies need to be designed in ways that include these factors for study. If we do not include hard-to-reach populations in the studies we cannot test for differences in relative risk reduction between easy to reach and hard to reach populations. As the authors note, disentangling the effects of risk factors in this way requires very large trials, something which researchers and research funding bodies have yet to address.

The problem of inconsistencies between the "intervention-focused" perspective of clinical epidemiology and the broader determinants of the health perspective of economics is not confined to the traditional territory of the clinical epidemiologist. The "intervention-focused" perspective has extended into the more traditional territory of the social sciences. For example, a recent Inquiry on Inequalities in Health in the UK population[26] produced a set of 39 "evidence-based" recommendations for changing the population distribution of health. Although research evidence was cited for most of these recommendations, none of this evidence related to the distribution of health in populations – precisely the focus of the Inquiry. The Inquiry focused attention on the "lower tail" of the health distribution, those with poor health, and recommendations ranged from "upstream" matters concerning the economic wellbeing of the poor to "downstream" matters concerning lifestyles and behaviours. In most cases the evidence presented in support of the recommendations was based on studies of interventions (including randomised trials) which did not report on the distribution of outcomes by social group. Moreover in some cases the studies were confined to non-poor subjects. Where poor subjects were studied, the outcomes measured (for example birth weight) were of limited value for drawing conclusions about either changes in health status or changes to the population distribution of health.[27]

What then are the messages for researchers concerned with improving the quality of the production and dissemination of research for decision makers? First, under the current restricted "intervention-focused" research paradigm several strategies could be pursued. Bias in study samples could be reduced by selecting a random sample of the population with the condition, subject to ethical considerations, as the focus of study. The information made available to decision makers by researchers should be presented in the context of a broader economic framework. This would include collecting and analysing information from a number of domains reflecting the broad determinants of health.

The extension of subgroup analyses could be employed to estimate differences in relative risk reduction by social group. However, subgroup analysis is based on a simple model of health production and assumptions that the different determinants of health are independent and separable. This fails to reflect the complex pathways to health in populations. The limitations of subgroup analyses could be addressed by employing advanced analytical techniques such as multilevel modelling[28] that better reflect the complex nature of health production. In this way we can move away from "evidence" about whether an intervention "works", a purposeful choice of the researcher potentially influenced by proprietary interests associated with the interventions.[29] Instead, research can be designed to generate information about the conditions under which particular interventions work best and whether the interventions selected for study work under the conditions experienced by those groups with greatest incidence or most need. Although these approaches would enrich the information base for decision makers, they remain constrained by an intervention focus. As a result, they are unable to find the "right" solution for the problems of populations but are more concerned with finding the right members of the population for the interventions. This biases attention in favour of better-off groups since they already have the advantage of greater exposure to other "non-clinical" determinants of health. Both the underlying frameworks for population health and the emerging empirical evidence suggest that better social conditions and social contexts are associated with better outcomes from interventions. Where the goal is to make best use of scarce health care resources this would imply giving priority to those who benefit most, better-off groups and a resulting increase in social inequalities in health.

An alternative strategy is to adopt a broader scientific paradigm together with research methods in which populations and their problems are the subject for study, and population heterogeneity is a source of information for the analysis, not a source of concern to be controlled.[10] The focus on evaluating interventions *per se* is replaced by understanding problems and identifying causes.[30] Population groups with the same health problems may be exposed to very different environments and hence have very different causes of that problem. The purposeful choices to be made concern which problems/settings to address as opposed to which interventions to study[31] and are, in principle, less affected by proprietary interests. Questions to be addressed include what is the problem, for whom is it a problem, why is it a problem and what is the impact of the problem? These questions will require a mixture of disciplinary approaches and analytical methods. Although this is unlikely to result in a rapidly expanding database of answers, that is a reflection of the complex nature of the society in which we live.

Until we adopt broader perspectives for policy-informing research, the use of the Cochrane database risks providing for decision makers what lampposts provide for drunks – support not illumination.

Summary points

- The Cochrane database is a collection of answers to questions posed by researchers about the impact of interventions on a health condition in a population.
- This provides information on whether an intervention works but not on the conditions under which an intervention works better or worse, or whether the intervention works in populations at greatest risk.
- Research methods used to provide answers deliberately control for these risk factors, which are distributed unequally in populations, and exclude "hard-to reach" populations, who are often at greatest risk.
- Health economics investigates the broad range of influences and constraints on the production of health, illness and recovery in populations.
- The incorporation of health economics into clinical studies has generally failed to utilise this broad conceptual basis and instead been constrained by the traditional confines of clinical epidemiology.
- This fails to reflect the complex pathways for the production of health, illness and recovery in populations and the social contexts in which problems faced by decision makers occur.
- Without information on the interface between social determinants of health and the impact of interventions, use of research findings can lead to decisions that reduce the efficiency of health care resource use and increase social inequalities in health.

References

1 Kerridge I, Lowe M, Henry D. Ethics and evidence based medicine. *BMJ* 1998;**316**:1151–3.
2 Chalmers I, Dickersin K, Chalmers TC. Getting to grips with Archie Cochrane's agenda. *BMJ* 1992;**305**:786–8.
3 Sackett DL, Rosenberg WM. On the need for evidence-based medicine. *Health Econ* 1995; **4**:249–54.

4 Sackett DL, Rosenberg WM. On the need for evidence-based medicine. *J Pub Health Med* 1995;**17**:330–4.
5 Jefferson T, Mugford M, Gray A, Demicheli V. An exercise on the feasibility of carrying out secondary economic analyses. *Health Econ* 1996;**5**:155–65.
6 Ham C, Hunter DJ, Robinson R. Evidence based policymaking. *BMJ* 1995;**310**:71–2.
7 Jefferson T, Demicheli V, Rivetti D, Deeks J. Cochrane reviews and systematic reviews of economic evaluations. Amantadine and rimantadine in the prevention and treatment of influenza. *Pharmacoeconomics* 1999;**16** (Suppl 1):85–9.
8 Haynes, RB, Sackett DL, Gray J, Muir A, Cook DJ, Guyatt GH. Transferring evidence from research into practice: 1. The role of clinical care research evidence in clinical decisions. *ACP Journal Club* 1996;**125**:A14.
9 Kothari A, Birch S. Concepts of rigour and implications for health services research. *J Health Serv Res Policy* 1998;**3**:121–3.
10 Birch S. As a matter of fact: evidence-based decision making unplugged. *Health Econ* 1997;**6**:547–59.
11 Ratcliffe JW, Gonzalez-del-Valle A. Rigor in health-related research: toward an expanded conceptualization. *Int J Health Serv* 1988;**18**:361–92.
12 Grossman M. The demand for health care: a theoretical and empirical investigation. *National Bureau of Economic Research Occasional Paper 119.* New York: Columbia University Press, 1972.
13 Evans RG, Stoddart GL. Producing health, consuming health care. *Soc Sci Med* 1990;**31**: 1347–63.
14 Hancock T. Lalonde and beyond: looking back at 'A new perspective on the health of Canadians'. *Health Prom* 1986;**1**:93–100.
15 Gunning-Schepers LJ, Hagen JH. Avoidable burden of illness: how much can prevention contribute to health? *Soc Sci Med* 1987;**24**:945–51.
16 Hurowitz JC. Toward a social policy for health. *N Engl J Med* 1993;**329**:130–3.
17 Lipworth L, Abelin T, Connelly RR. Socioeconomic factors in the prognosis of cancer patients. *J Chron Dis* 1970;**23**:105–15.
18 Leon D, Wilkinson R. Social inequalities in prognosis. In: Fox J, Carr-Hill R, eds. *Health Inequalities in European Countries.* Aldershot: Gower, 1989.
19 Carnon AG, Ssemwogerere A, Lamont DW, Hole DJ, Mallon EA, George WD *et al.* Relation between socioeconomic deprivation and pathological prognostic factors in women with breast cancer. *BMJ* 1994;**309**:1054–7.
20 Alter DA, Naylor CD, Austin P, Tu JV. Effects of socioeconomic status on access to invasive cardiac procedures and on mortality after acute myocardial infarction. *N Engl J Med* 1999; **341**:1359–67.
21 Sackett DL, Rosenberg WM, Gray JA, Haynes RB, Richardson WS. Evidence based medicine: what it is and what it isn't. *BMJ* 1996;**312**:71–2.
22 Simpson E. The interpretation of interactions in contingency tables. *J R Stat Soc* 1951;**13**: 238–41.
23 Utts J. *Seeing through statistics.* Toronto: Duxbury, 1996.
24 Haynes RB, Taylor DW, Sackett DL, Thorpe K, Ferguson GG, Barnett HJ. Prevention of functional impairment by endarterectomy for symptomatic high-grade carotid stenosis. North American Symptomatic Carotid Endarterectomy Trial Collaborators. *JAMA* 1994;**271**:1256–9.
25 Glasziou PP, Irwig LM. An evidence based approach to individualising treatment. *BMJ* 1995; **311**:1356–9.
26 Acheson D, Barker D, Cambers J *et al.* Independent Inquiry into Inequalities in Health Report. London: The Stationery Office, 1998.
27 Birch S. The 39 steps: the mystery of health inequalities in the UK. *Health Econ* 1999;**8**:301–8.
28 Rice N, Jones A. Multilevel models and health economics. *Health Econ* 1997;**6**:561–75.
29 Morgan S, Barer M, Evans R. Health economists meet the fourth tempter: drug dependency and scientific discourse. *Health Econ* 2000;**9**:659–67.
30 Syme SL. Social and economic disparities in health: thoughts about intervention. *Milbank Q* 1998;**76**:493–7.
31 Oakley A. Who cares for health? Social relations, gender, and the public health. Duncan Memorial Lecture. *J Epidemiol Community Health* 1994;**48**:427–34.

11: Evidence-based medicine meets economic evaluation – an agenda for research

MICHAEL DRUMMOND

Introduction

Any nuclear physicist could tell us that, when different particles come together, there will be either fusion or fission! The attempt, through this book, to merge some of the key concepts of evidence-based medicine (EBM) and economic evaluation is based on the premise that there is considerable scope for fusion. The outcome suggests that, indeed, the scope for fusion is substantial, but that it is not without a modicum of fission.

This chapter explores the following issues:

- In what ways can the approaches embodied in EBM support, or enhance, the work of those conducting economic evaluations?
- In what ways are the approaches embodied in EBM unhelpful, or even counterproductive, when viewed from an economic perspective?
- In the interests of greater fusion in the future, what are the priorities for further research?

In the next section the use of systematic reviews in economic evaluation is discussed. The problems of conducting systematic reviews of economic evaluation are then explored and the difficulties in obtaining evidence about broader (non-clinical) health policies and interventions are outlined. Finally, a number of topics for further research are identified and a few conclusions drawn.

Using systematic reviews in economic evaluation

Estimates of the effectiveness of medical interventions are a critical feature of economic evaluations. In an ideal world the estimate of effectiveness used in an economic study should be internally valid (that is, free from bias) and externally valid (that is, generalisable to other settings). However, several reviews of economic evaluation[1,2] indicate that the incorporation of poor effectiveness evidence is a common weakness in published studies and some authors have also pointed to the potential for bias when an economic evaluation uses a subset of the available clinical data.[3,4]

Therefore, there is a strong *prima facie* case for using the estimates of effect size from systematic reviews as an input to economic evaluations. Certainly they provide a more precise and less biased estimate than that obtained from a single clinical study. Whether or not the output of systematic reviews satisfies the need for external validity in economic evaluations is less clear. In part this depends on whether the effect size of medical interventions varies greatly from setting to setting. Often it may not, in which case the summary estimate from a systematic review will be relevant for a range of settings. However, if it does vary it might be better to use, in an economic evaluation, the estimate of effect size most relevant to the setting in which the economic evaluation is being performed.

The other potential concern in using the estimate of effect size from systematic reviews in economic evaluations arises, paradoxically, from the main methodological strength of such reviews. That is, systematic reviews usually rely heavily on data from randomised controlled trials (RCTs), as the criteria for the inclusion of studies in the review usually exclude non-random studies or case series. Whilst this makes a lot of sense, there could be a threat to external validity owing to the fact that many RCTs are undertaken under conditions atypical of regular clinical practice; that is, they are designed to assess efficacy rather than effectiveness.[5,6] However, faced with a choice of lower internal validity (through the inclusion of poorly controlled studies), or lower external validity (through an emphasis on randomised controlled trials), most economists would still opt for the latter.[7]

Several chapters in this book address issues associated with the use of data from systematic reviews in economic evaluation. The contributions from Mugford, and Farquhar and Brown in Chapters 3 and 4 illustrate very clearly the advantages of basing economic evaluations on systematic reviews. Chapter 5, by Coyle and Lee, demonstrates how the results of economic evaluations are critically dependent on the data sources, including the estimate of clinical effect size. They also show how widely the cost-effectiveness of an intervention can vary when estimates of effect size are taken from individual trials, as opposed to the systematic review.

Therefore, whereas the outputs of systematic reviews of clinical studies are clearly very useful for those undertaking economic evaluations, economists need to think carefully about how the estimates of effect size should be interpreted. In addition, there may be ways in which the selection of studies, their critical appraisal and presentation could be modified in order to make the outputs of systematic reviews even more useful to those undertaking economic evaluations.[8]

Undertaking systematic reviews of economic evaluations

If the outputs of systematic reviews of clinical studies are a useful data source for economic evaluations, can the methodology of systematic review be applied to the economic evaluations themselves?

The great advantage of systematic reviews of clinical studies is that they produce authoritative estimates of the effect size of medical interventions, based on a careful selection, and critical appraisal, of the existing literature. It would be tempting to think that, by a careful identification and review of economic evaluations of a given intervention, we could make similarly authoritative statements about whether "therapy X is cost-effective".

The contributions to this book by Mugford (Chapter 3), Coyle and Lee (Chapter 5), Jefferson *et al* (Chapter 6), Demicheli *et al* (Chapter 7) and Ament *et al* (Chapter 8) suggest that we may be some distance from reaching this position. The first problem is that the methodology of published economic evaluations appears to be unstandardised, at least when compared with the methodology of clinical trials. This lack of standardisation has arisen, apparently, in spite of all the efforts to propose guidelines for the methodology of economic studies. It can perhaps be understood in situations where the guidelines are fairly general, such as those produced by the BMJ Working Party on Economic Evaluation.[9] However, lack of standardisation and methodological shortcomings are also found in situations where the guidelines are quite specific, such as in the guidelines for submissions to the Pharmaceutical Benefits Advisory Committee in Australia.[10]

The second problem relates to a lack of agreement on quality standards for economic evaluations. The published guidelines imply general quality standards. For example, the BMJ Working Party guidelines have a checklist of 31 items.[9] However, there is no clear indication of which items are the most important, nor which items would be critical to the inclusion of a particular economic evaluation in a systematic review. That is, there appear to be no primary criteria for a good economic evaluation that would be analogous to those used to judge the quality of clinical studies; for example, random assignment of patients to treatment groups, concealment of assignment to both patient and physician, and so on.

Thirdly, it is not clear that the motivation to produce an authoritative statement of cost-effectiveness is as strong as it appears to be for statements of clinical effect size. This is because there is widespread recognition amongst economists, and possibly amongst decision makers, that whether or not a particular intervention is cost-effective depends on the local situation. Indeed, several authors have identified the factors that may affect the cost-effectiveness of interventions. These include the basic demography and epidemiology of disease, relative price levels, availability of health care resources and clinical practice patterns and conventions.[11,12]

Therefore, the real contribution of a systematic review of economic evaluations may not be to produce a single authoritative result, but to help decision makers understand the structure of the resource allocation problem they are addressing and the impact, on the overall result, of the main parameters. Thus, the emphasis in such a review is likely to be less on producing a summarised estimate of the cost-effectiveness ratio, and more on demonstrating by how much this varies from setting to setting, and why it varies. Nevertheless, economists could still learn a considerable amount from the methodology of systematic review, including the need to be meticulous in searching the published and unpublished literature, and the need to devise explicit inclusion and exclusion criteria for studies.

Obtaining evidence about the effects of broader health policies and interventions

A central tenet of EBM is the primacy of the RCT as the method for estimating the effect size of medical interventions. The same logic extends to systematic review to assess effectiveness of health interventions, since the inclusion criteria for studies favour RCTs. However, whilst acknowledging the importance of the RCT for assessing medical interventions, Chapters 9 and 10 in this book (by Kristiansen and Gosden, and Birch) raise a number of questions about its relevance to the evaluation of broader health policies and interventions.

First, evidence from RCTs may not be available for some programmes and policies (Kristiansen and Gosden discuss this in the context of payment systems for primary care providers). Whereas in some cases the lack of RCTs may reflect the lack of imagination or methodological rigour of those undertaking the research, in others it may reflect the fact that it is difficult or impractical to carry out controlled experiments. The reasons for this are several and include: (i) the difficulties of maintaining blinding in studies, especially where subjects need information in order to respond to incentives/disincentives; (ii) doubts about the external validity of study findings, given the artificial nature of trials; and (iii) political sensitivities about the use of randomised designs in assessing public policy measures.

For example, an "evidence-based" evaluation of Health Action Zones (HAZs) in the UK would require us to identify a sample of geographical areas likely to benefit and then to randomise a proportion to receive HAZ funding and a proportion not. Then, after several years, it would be possible to make an assessment of the costs and benefits of the policy. There are several examples of RCTs of social policy interventions.[13] However, whether such an approach would always be politically feasible is another matter.

These problems suggest that the results of observational studies should have more emphasis in systematic reviews. If this were the case, more thought would need to be given to developing criteria for assessing the methodological quality of observational studies. However, the chapter by Kristiansen and Gosden outlines some of the problems in doing this, and the threats to internal validity that arise when non-randomised studies are used.

In his chapter, Birch raises some more fundamental criticisms of the approaches embodied in EBM, including the randomised controlled trial. However, rather than merely suggesting that the RCT is inappropriate or impractical in some situations, he argues that in some circumstances it may be positively misleading or counterproductive.

In particular, he argues that the RCT produces an average result for all those enrolled in the trial, whereas often one is interested in the impact of health policies on particular subgroups of the population. In addition, he argues that, unavoidably, the results of many health policies are context-specific and that the "cleansing" of problems that is necessary to conduct experiments like RCTs inevitably means that some of this context is lost.

Finally, the focus on RCTs may bias the research agenda towards the study of interventions (particularly medical ones) that are more easily evaluated in this way. This will cause economists to be diverted from exploring aspects of the broader determinants of health, which may be more fundamental to improving the health of the population.

Many of Birch's comments lead us back to the inevitable trade-off, in conducting research, between internal and external validity. The traditional EBM approach, focusing on RCTs, has high internal validity. The central question is whether it can be modified to take account of these criticisms, without sacrificing too many of its advantages.

For example, several RCTs have been conducted with a more pragmatic design, enrolling a broader patient population and being conducted under "real life" conditions.[14] However, they are more difficult to conduct and to analyse. It is also possible to accommodate subgroup analysis in the design of RCTs, or to perform statistical analyses of the results to explore some of the demographic influences that Birch alludes to.

In some cases it may be necessary, as Birch suggests, to move to a different paradigm. However, this has its disadvantages too. The concerns that Birch raises about the discretion analysts have in the design of experiments (and hence the simplification of the problem) merely transfer to concerns about the discretion researchers would have in the interpretation of the results of studies that have several threats to internal validity. Perhaps we need both approaches, so as to balance one set of concerns against the other.

A research agenda

Given the issues identified above, what research should be undertaken in order to increase the potential for fusion between EBM and economic evaluation? Some suggestions are given below.

Systematic reviews of clinical studies

In order to increase the usefulness, for economic evaluation, of systematic reviews of clinical studies, it would be of interest to answer the following questions:

- In what ways should the inclusion criteria for studies in systematic reviews be modified to accommodate the needs of economic evaluation?
- Can quality criteria be developed for non-randomised, or observational, studies?
- How can non-RCT data best be incorporated in systematic reviews?
- Is it possible, or desirable, for systematic reviews to give an estimate of the clinical effect size for subgroups of the patient population, as well as the average effect size?
- How can issues of external validity (generalisability) be better addressed in systematic reviews of clinical studies?

Systematic review, and critical appraisal, of economic evaluations

More exploration is required of whether it is possible, or desirable, to undertake systematic reviews of economic studies. In particular, it would be useful to answer the following questions:

- What are the possible objectives in undertaking systematic reviews of economic evaluations and are these attainable?
- Can the *really critical* methodological features of economic evaluations be identified, so as to guide decisions on the inclusion of studies in systematic reviews?
- Can a quality score (or grading) system be developed for economic evaluations, and how would such a system be validated?

Evaluation of broader health interventions

Whilst the "standard" RCT methodology is normally the preferred approach for evaluating medical interventions, the evaluation of other, broader, health interventions may require different approaches. The extent to which this is the case could be assessed by answering the following questions:

- What are the real (*and imagined!*) problems of conducting RCTs of policy measures?
- Would more pragmatic designs for clinical trials address some of the concerns about unnecessary simplification of problems and increase the practical relevance of study results?
- In which situations would RCTs *not* be the preferred approach and can these situations be easily identified?
- Can we define more clearly the limits of the EBM paradigm and specify more fully the alternatives?

Conclusions

This meeting of evidence-based medicine and economic evaluation suggests that, overall, there is more fusion than fission. In particular, the outputs of systematic reviews of clinical studies are useful for economic evaluation and some of the methodologies embodied in systematic reviews (that is, literature search, critical appraisal of studies) could usefully be adopted by those undertaking economic studies.

However, some of the methodologies of EBM require modification in order to maximise their full potential for economic evaluation and some may not be useful at all.

On balance, further dialogue between those involved in EBM and economic evaluation will add more than it subtracts. Nevertheless, economists would do well to cast a critical eye on EBM methodologies and should not adopt them without careful thought. Advocates of EBM would expect nothing less.

References

1 Udvarhelyi IS, Colditz GA, Rai A, Epstein AM. Cost-effectiveness and cost-benefit analyses in the medical literature. Are the methods being used correctly? *Ann Intern Med* 1992;**116**:238–44.
2 Elixhauser A, Halpern M, Schmier J, Luce BR. Health care CBA and CEA from 1991 to 1996: an updated bibliography. *Med Care* 1998;**36**:MS1–147.
3 Freemantle N, Maynard A. Something rotten in the state of clinical and economic evaluations? *Health Econ* 1994;**3**:63–7.
4 Jönsson B. Economic evaluation and clinical uncertainty: response to Freemantle and Maynard. *Health Econ* 1994;**3**:305–7.
5 Drummond MF. *Economic analysis alongside controlled trials: an introduction for clinical researchers*. London: Department of Health, 1994.
6 O'Brien B. Economical evaluation of pharmaceuticals: Frankenstein's monster or vampire of trials? *Med Care* 1996;**34**:DS99–108.
7 Drummond MF. Experimental versus observational data in the economic evaluation of pharmaceuticals. *Med Decision Making* 1998;**18**:S12–18.
8 Pang F, Drummond MF, Song F. *The use of meta-analysis in economic evaluation*. Centre for Health Economics Discussion Paper 173. University of York, 1999.
9 Drummond M, Jefferson T and the BMJ Economic Evaluation Working Party. Guidelines for authors and peer reviewers of economic submissions to the BMJ. *BMJ* 1996;**313**:275–83.
10 Hill SR, Mitchell AS, Henry DA. Problems with the interpretation of pharmacoeconomic analyses: a review of submissions to the Australian Pharmaceutical Benefits Scheme. *JAMA* 2000;**283**:2116–21.
11 Drummond MF, Bloom BS, Carrin G, Hillman AL, Hutchings HC, Knill-Jones RP *et al.* Issues in the cross-national assessment of health technology. *Int J Technol Assess Health Care* 1992;**8**:671–82.
12 Koopmanschap MA, Touw KCR, Rutten FFH. Analysis of costs and cost-effectiveness in multinational trials. *Health Policy* 2001;**58**:175–86.
13 Oakley A. *Experiments in knowing*. Cambridge: Polity Press, 2000.
14 Drummond MF, Knapp MRJ, Burns TP, Miller KD, Shadwell P. Issues in the design of studies for the economic evaluation of a new, atypical antipsychotic: the ESTO Study. *J Ment Health Policy Econ* 1998;**1**:15–22.

12: Glossary of terms for health economics and systematic review

GILLIAN CURRIE, BRADEN MANNS

Administrative data consists of data sets that can be used to assess the "real world" prevalence and incidence of disease and/or use of health care resources.

Allocative efficiency refers to decisions about the distribution of health care resources across health care programmes, that is how much, or whether, to invest resources in a particular health care programme versus another. In contrast to **technical efficiency**, when a decision of this type is made, one group of patients gains at the expense of another. Allocative efficiency occurs when the outcomes achieved with the available resources match the priorities of society.

Benefits of a health care intervention include health outcomes, effects on wellbeing not related to the health impact *per se* (for example, information or reassurance) and production gains. Offsetting these positive impacts on the benefit side are negative impacts such as health deterioration (due to adverse effects), effects on wellbeing not related to the health impact (such as anxiety) and production losses.

Bias refers to a systematic error in the design or conduct of a research study that results in a distortion of the inferences made from the data. It may be intentional or accidental.

Capitation is a method of remuneration in which providers are given a fixed payment based on the number of patients under their care; payments are not dependent upon the amount of medical treatments or services provided.

Checklists are a means of assessing the quality of a completed study, which incorporates the extent to which existing **guidelines** are followed, whereby a set of criteria used to assess the quality of a study are listed and possibly prioritised.

Confounding occurs when there is a variable that can affect the outcome of interest which is associated with the one or more of the factors being investigated. If it cannot be adjusted for, the effect of the confounding variables may be indistinguishable from the factors being studied, rendering it impossible to draw conclusions about the causal relationship of the factors under investigation on the outcome of interest.

Conjoint analysis is a technique for valuing the benefits of health services by asking respondents to make discrete choices between alternative bundles of attributes which make up that health service. If the cost of the service is one of the included attributes, this technique allows one to determine **willingness to pay** indirectly.

Contingent valuation is a technique for valuing the benefits of health services, typically by determining individuals' maximum **willingness to pay** for the availability of that health service or the minimum amount they would accept as compensation for not having that service available.

Costs refer to the value of any resources that have an **opportunity cost** as a result of being used in that health care service, in the context of an economic evaluation of a health care service or intervention.

Cost-benefit analysis is a form of economic evaluation whereby all the costs and benefits are included and used to address the **allocative efficiency** question of whether a particular health care service is worthwhile. In a full cost-benefit analysis, all benefits are valued in monetary terms (using techniques to assess **willingness to pay** such as **contingent valuation** or **conjoint analysis**) and thus the costs and benefits can be directly compared to assess whether the project is worthwhile.

Cost-consequence analysis is a partial economic evaluation whereby an array of health outcome measures are enumerated alongside costs. This is distinct from **cost-effectiveness analysis** where there is a single health outcome measure. In cost-consequence analysis, an overall valuation of the bundle of health outcome measures is not attempted but rather left to the decision maker. Thus, it may be viewed as a partial **cost-benefit analysis**.

Cost-effectiveness acceptability curve is a graphical representation of the percentage of replications within a simulation exercise where the **incremental cost-effectiveness ratio** is below a specific threshold.

Cost-effectiveness analysis is a form of economic evaluation that addresses questions of **technical efficiency**. Comparisons are limited to services or treatment options that produce the same type of benefit which is valued strictly in one-dimensional, naturally occurring units.

Cost of illness studies aim to identify and measure the total costs attributable to a particular disease. These are not a type of **economic evaluation**, as they are not used to assess the **costs** and **benefits** of alternative courses of action. They may provide useful information which can be used in the context of an economic evaluation of interventions related to the disease category, although care must be taken as not all costs included in a cost of illness study represent resource costs.

Cost-minimisation analysis is a special type of **cost-effectiveness analysis** which is possible only if it has been determined that there is no difference in benefits between two alternative interventions and thus the evaluation can be made based upon costs alone.

Cost per QALY is a way of expressing the results of a **cost-utility analysis**, in terms of a cost per unit of benefit attained which is measured in **quality-adjusted life years (QALYs)**.

Cost-utility analysis is a variant of **cost-effectiveness analysis** where the health outcome measure of interest is usually expressed as a **quality-adjusted life year**, which is a single index that combines length of life and a quality adjustment for less than perfect health states (that is, the **utility** score).

Decision analysis is a systematic approach to decision making under conditions of uncertainty. It is used to determine the **costs** and health outcomes for a hypothetical patient cohort with the disease of interest when they are treated with different clinical strategies. The analysis may incorporate information derived from observational data sets that provide information on prevalence, average mortality rates and costs, or from clinical trials that examine the effectiveness of a therapy.

A **Delphi panel** is a structured group communication method designed to reach consensus, if possible, on particular issues. Thus, it provides a means of synthesizing information from a wide range of sources, particularly from unpublished material via experts.

The **determinants of health** refer to the various inputs to the production of health in a population, including medical care, socioeconomic factors, environment, genetics and individual behaviour.

Discounting is the process of converting **costs** or **benefits** to be incurred or received at different points in the future to a present value so that they can be compared in commensurate units as if they all occurred at the same point in time.

Ecological fallacy refers to the potential to draw incorrect inferences on individual level associations on the basis of aggregate level associations. (For example, aggregate data may indicate an association between fee-for-service payment and use of laboratory tests although there is no effect of payment system on the likelihood of ordering tests at an individual consultation.)

Economic evaluation is the application of analytical methods to identify, measure and value both the **costs** and **benefits** of alternative health care interventions in order to provide evidence regarding **technical** or **allocative efficiency** and aid decision making for resource allocation.

Effect size is a measure of the difference in effect between intervention and control treatments. This may measure the absolute difference in the means or proportions, or may be a standardised measure taking account of variance of the mean and size of sample.

Effectiveness refers to the extent to which a given intervention or service produces health outcomes in individuals who are offered that intervention or service. This will be dependent on both the **efficacy** of the treatment, but also the acceptance and compliance with the treatment in "real world" environments.

Efficacy refers to the extent to which a given intervention or service produces a particular health outcome in individuals who fully comply with the recommended treatment under ideal clinical settings. This is in contrast to **effectiveness**.

Efficiency refers to making the optimal use of scarce resources. There are two (related) types of efficiency: **technical** and **allocative** efficiency.

Epidemiology is a field of study that examines the statistical frequency, distribution and determinants of disease in a population and evaluates the clinical effectiveness of different forms of care. The latter is sometimes referred to as Health Services Research. This field is important for health economists by providing information on disease prevalence, natural history of disease etc.

Evidence-based medicine describes the systematic and rigorous use of methods to evaluate existing clinical studies, in order to deliver best clinical care to individuals or groups of patients. It includes the following steps:

asking a relevant clinical question, performing a target-oriented literature search, critically appraising the literature using established guidelines, and attempting to apply the gained information to clinical practice.

External validity refers to the extent to which the results of a study can be transferred to another patient group that is different from the original group of patients studied.

Fee-for-service is a method of remuneration by which health providers are given payment in return for specific medical treatment.

Financial incentive refers to the potential to influence professionals' behaviour, either by affecting their income or their expenditure related to alternative decisions.

Generalisability of results is similar to **external validity** in that it refers to the extent to which information (both clinical and economic) can be extrapolated to either a patient group with different characteristics or to a similar patient group treated in a different geographic, political or time structure. See also **transferability**.

Guidelines refer to statements that reflect the suggested course or procedure to follow and are meant to be based on best current evidence.

Health economics is the study of the economic aspects of health and health care. It combines methods and theories from traditional economics and epidemiology and can serve as an important supplement to the routine clinical information used by medical and health care programmes.

Health technology assessment is the systematic evaluation of the properties, effects and/or other impacts of health care technology. It is designed to provide objective information to support health care decisions and policy making.

Health-related quality of life (HRQOL) refers to the physical, social and emotional aspects that are relevant and important to a patient's wellbeing. It can be assessed using a disease-specific, generic or a preference-based measurement tool.

Healthy year equivalents (HYE) refers to the hypothetical number of years spent in perfect health that could be considered equivalent to a defined number of years spent in a certain state of imperfect health. Similar to QALYs, it attempts to measure a person's preference for a particular health state. Unlike QALYs, it measures preference over an entire continuous path of defined health states.

Incremental cost-effectiveness ratio: From the results of a cost-effectiveness analysis an **incremental cost-effectiveness ratio** can be calculated that depicts the extra cost per unit of outcome obtained, in comparing one treatment option to another. In this case, a value judgement will be required to assess whether the extra unit of outcome is worthwhile (see **cost-benefit analysis**).

Internal validity refers to whether the results obtained from a study are valid and true for the group of patients that were treated within a specific trial. Sources of **bias** (including **selection bias**) should be minimised to enhance the internal validity of a study. Guidelines have been developed (namely the JAMA Users' Guide to the Medical Literature) to enable readers of clinical trials to determine whether the studies have any features that threaten internal validity.

Markov model: Within this type of **modelling** patients with a specific clinical problem can exist in a finite set of health states (that is: alive in perfect health, alive with a deficit in HRQOL, or dead) between which they can move over time. Movement between these health states occurs over a discrete time interval, usually yearly (known as a Markov cycle) based on preset transition probabilities. By attaching resource costs and health outcome consequences to each Markov state (which may vary based on use of an intervention), it is possible to test how such an intervention might influence clinical outcomes and resource use (on average) for a group of patients with a clinical problem.

Meta-analysis is a quantitative form of **systematic review** consisting of searching for, evaluating and combining numerically the results of relevant studies that examine the effect of the same intervention on a defined outcome to derive an overall estimate of the clinical effect.

Modelling is a tool used by health economists to determine the most likely health outcome and resource consequences of choosing to use an intervention to treat a hypothetical cohort of patients with a defined clinical condition. It often involves the use of **decision analysis**.

Monte Carlo simulation is used in **decision analysis**. It uses simulation methods to simultaneously deal with the potential uncertainty surrounding each important clinical or costing variable. In this method, each transition probability, clinical outcome or cost is represented as a variable quantity with a range of possible values described by a probability distribution function. Such a function simply gives the probabilities that the variable concerned equals each of a sequence of possible values.

Observational studies are non-intervention studies (usually case-control or cohort studies) that usually examine the effect of exposure to risk factors on specified health outcomes.

Opportunity cost, a concept central to health economics, rests on two principles: scarcity of resources and choice. Due to the presence of scarcity of resources, society must make choices about what health programmes to fund and which ones to forgo. It is the benefits that are associated with forgone health care programmes or opportunities that constitute opportunity costs.

Primary studies are studies that rely on original data to answer study questions.

Quality-adjusted life year (QALY) is a measure of health outcome which incorporates the effect of an intervention on both length of life and the quality of life. QALYs are calculated by multiplying the total years gained through use of a specific treatment (or the number of life years remaining) by the "utility" of those years (measured from zero, representing the worst imaginable health, to 1, representing perfect health).

Randomised controlled trial (RCT) is an experimental study design in which the intervention is randomly allocated to study participants.

Resources refer to all the components that are used in the production of a good or service. Within health care, resources refer not only to financial resources, but also to other resources such as doctors, nurses, buildings, equipment and supplies.

Selection bias refers to systematic differences between comparison groups in prognosis or responsiveness to treatment, resulting from the manner in which subjects are selected. Random allocation with adequate concealment of allocation protects against selection bias. Biases resulting from studying an unrepresentative sample of the population are covered under **generalisability**.

Sensitivity analysis is a technique used in **economic evaluation** or **decision analysis** to determine how and/or whether plausible changes in uncertain clinical or costing variables affect the main results of the analysis.

Systematic review refers to the application of explicit methods to comprehensive identification, as well as subsequent review and either a qualitative or a quantitative synthesis of all the literature on a specific topic, usually using a defined search strategy and reporting framework. When the results of studies can be combined quantitatively using appropriate statistical methodology, rather than in just a qualitative fashion, this is usually termed a **meta-analysis**.

Technical efficiency: Within economics, technical efficiency refers to the production of the maximum level of output for a certain combination of input factors (that is, raw material, working hours etc). Within health care, it usually refers to how to deliver a programme or to achieve a given objective with the fewest resources. In general, with technical efficiency, the same group will be treated to achieve a certain outcome, the question being by which method.

Transferability refers to the ability to extrapolate results obtained from one setting or context to another. See also **generalisability**

Utility is a measure of the preference for a specific health outcome. A utility can be derived from a direct measurement approach (such as a standard gamble or time trade-off exercise) or from a preference-based scale (the best known being the Health Utilities Index or Euroqol EQ-5D). All approaches result in a number from zero, representing the worst imaginable health, to one, representing perfect health, and can be directly incorporated into **QALYs** for use in **economic evaluations**.

Viewpoint refers to the perspective of the likely readers and users of the economic evaluation. Analyses can be done from the perspective of the health care provider (in which case patient-related expenses such as time off work due to illness are ignored), society (in which case all costs/benefits are considered, regardless of to whom they accrue), a medical insurer or the patient. As suggested, the analyses differ with respect to what costs and benefits are considered.

Willingness to pay (WTP) is a technique that is used to measure preferences for benefits of health services or interventions in monetary terms. In this method, the maximum amount of money an individual is willing to pay to gain a particular benefit (that is, receive a certain health care intervention) is elicited by direct questioning.

Index

Page numbers in **bold** type refer to figures; those in *italic* refer to tables or boxed material